A Missy Barrett Chapter Book

I0408268

PINWHEELS
and
PEARLS

ELYSE BRUCE

PINWHEELS AND PEARLS

CHAPTER 1

Nine year old Missy Barrett sat quietly in the passenger seat of her Grandma Barrett's fancy car. Usually Missy had lots to talk about when she and her grandmother went somewhere together, but today was different. Today, Missy was noticing a number of yard signs she hadn't seen before, and they were all the same.

There was a purple star in the top corner, and a purple crescent moon just below it. That was on the left side of the picture. On the right side were three purple triangles, then three purple words: *Relay For Life*. Underneath that, was a red and blue logo. There were other things written on the signs but the car was moving, so it was hard to read everything quickly. Instead, Missy focused on the pretty picture as she wondered what *Relay For Life* meant.

"You're awfully quiet over there," Grandma Barrett finally said.

"I'm just trying to figure something out," Missy replied as they drove past another sign.

"Sometimes when I'm trying to figure something out, I'll ask your grandpa what he thinks," her grandma said helpfully.

"I would ask grandpa if he was here," Missy replied politely, "but he's not here. It's just the two of us, Grandma."

Grandma Barrett chuckled quietly to herself. She hadn't meant that Missy should ask her grandpa for advice. She was hoping that Missy might tell *her* what she was thinking.

"I know, sweetie," Grandma Barrett said. "I guess you'll just have to make do with me."

Missy turned her head towards her grandma. "I'm sorry, Grandma," she apologized. "I didn't mean you couldn't help. I was just busy thinking about the signs so I wasn't thinking about my words."

"That's all right," Grandma Barrett assured Missy. "Sometimes I say things without thinking. It's a people thing. I'm not upset."

Missy breathed a sigh of relief. She was happy to hear her grandma wasn't hurt by her comment. She looked back out the window, then asked, "What's a *Relay For Life*?"

"What's a what?"

"A *Relay For Life*," Missy repeated. "What is it?"

"Well, I imagine it's a race of some sort," Grandma Barrett replied, "but I don't know what the *For Life* part would be all about."

"Do you think Grandpa knows what it means?" Missy asked. Looking at her grandma's purse that sat between the two of them on the armrest, Missy pondered whether she should ask permission to get her grandma's cellphone out so she could call her grandpa.

"I imagine he might," Grandma Barrett replied. "He knows about those sorts of things." She paused. "Of course, sometimes he doesn't, but what he doesn't know, he's good at finding out. He's been that way since before we met."

"And that was in the old-fashioned days, right?" Missy interrupted, her eyes twinkling with mischief. "It was back in the day when going out on a date with a boy meant you were going to share a chocolate milkshake at the diner. That's what they always do in the black-and-white movies from the old-fashioned days."

"Your grandpa never made us share a chocolate milkshake. When we went out on a date, he always had money for his own milkshake," Grandma Barrett said with a laugh.

"Didn't Grandpa like sharing, Grandma?"

"It wasn't about sharing or not sharing," her grandma explained. "Your grandpa made sure he had enough money so we could each have our own milkshake. That's how your grandpa won my heart."

"One milkshake at a time," Missy sighed as she imagined her grandma as a young teenager being swept off her feet by a dashing young teenage grandpa. The pretend scene continued to play out in Missy's mind for a few seconds before she asked, "Do you think boys will buy *me* my very own chocolate milkshake when I'm old enough to go out on a date?"

"I'm pretty sure they will, Missy, but that's a long way off from now," her grandma guaranteed her.

"A *really* long way off according to Aaron and Josh," Missy confessed, "and a really, *really* long way off if you ask mom."

Aaron and Josh were Missy's older brothers. Josh was attending high school, and Aaron was already in college, and together with their mom, Jenna, they lived in a small house that was built around the time Grandma and Grandpa Barrett were children in grade school.

"And an even *longer* way off if you were to ask your grandpa," her grandmother joked. The car slowed as grandma pulled into the parking lot, and Missy peered through the windshield to see if she could find a spot for her grandmother.

"There's one right in front of Cassie's front door," she pointed out excitedly. She clapped her hands. She was thrilled she was going to have her hair trimmed by her favorite hair stylist.

"Hey, you know what else, Grandma?" Missy asked. "Maybe Cassie or Mackie or Christin know lots of stuff about *Relay For Life*. We should ask them!"

Missy's grandma smiled at her granddaughter. Missy made it a point to learn as many details as possible about new things that interested her. There was no doubt in Grandma Barrett's mind that finding out about *Relay For Life* wasn't a passing fancy. After all, Missy loved telling people: If you're brought to it, you've got to go do it.

Grandma Barrett turned the car off.

"Remember to be on your best behavior, Missy," her grandmother reminded her. "This is a place of business. It's not a playground even if they *do* have hula hoops."

"I promise," Missy agreed. Checking first to make sure it was safe to open the door, Missy was certain as she stepped out of the car that someone at Shear Madness would know something about *Relay For Life*.

CHAPTER 2

While Missy's brothers moaned and groaned each time Monday morning rolled around, Missy loved Mondays. Monday meant the start of a new week, and that meant adventures were waiting for her somewhere out there.

This morning, all the classes had been called to the gym for an Assembly. That's what the principal called it when everyone went to the gym for a special announcement. Missy wondered what the big surprise might be. Maybe the school had won an award. Maybe it was something like the Nobel Peace Prize for best-behaved school. Maybe it was to reveal the school had taken first prize in the television show *Smartest Students*.

Sitting quietly on the gym floor with her classmates, Missy did a visual inspection of the stage hoping to find clues. The stage wasn't a stage the way most people thought of stages.

Missy had stood on the stage once before when she won a special award. To her way of thinking, it was like four tables smooshed up together with a carpet across them, and a two-step ladder like what her Grandma Barrett had in her kitchen at either end. Along the front were black, pleated drapes that were stuck to the tables with heavy plastic clips so they could be removed and put away later.

Just like the drapery, the stage could also be broken down so it was as flat as possible, taking into consideration the table legs. Missy worried whenever the stage was up, mostly because she thought it might collapse although it never had before. But she couldn't shake that worry. Perhaps it was because her mother didn't like her or her brothers standing on the picnic table in the backyard, and Missy thought it was probably because the table might collapse with all that added weight.

But this wasn't made out of wood like their picnic table, Missy reasoned, so perhaps when tables were made out of steel, they were much safer to stand on.

Sometimes there was a podium on the stage, but most of the time, it was just a microphone on a stand, and the cable was secured with silver-colored tape holding it down so no one would trip over it if they were on the stage.

Excited voices washed across the gym as teachers tried to hush and calm their classes, some with gentle nods and others with stern looks. Missy knew the faster everyone quieted down, the sooner the principal would take to the stage to share the news.

The door at the far end of the gym opened, and the school principal, followed by four strangers, entered. They strode over to the stage, walked up the two steps, and stood before everyone. The principal stood behind the microphone, and the strangers stood to her left.

"Good morning students," the principal said cheerily. Missy could tell that whatever the principal was going to share, it was going to be wonderful news. She could hear it in the tone and timber of her voice.

"Good morning, Mrs. Mahoney," the student body replied in unison.

"We have some guests with us today, and I expect you to give them the respect you give me when I speak," Mrs. Mahoney told everyone. "Today we'll be hearing about *Relay For Life* and how our school can help save lives."

Missy clapped her hands together loudly, and her classmates joined in as much out of surprise as because they thought perhaps this *was* the time to applaud the principal. Perhaps it wasn't, but Missy hadn't thought about that. All she knew was that whatever Mrs. Mahoney had planned, it was going to save lives, and the entire student body was going to help.

"Today we have some very special guests with us," Mrs. Mahoney continued once the applause quieted down. "I'd like to introduce Ms. Conerly from *Relay For Life*."

A tall woman with blond hair and a big smile waved at the students.

"Mrs. Bowman."

The woman standing next to Ms. Conerly also waved at the students.

"Dr. Dodge," Mrs. Mahoney continued. Dr. Dodge nodded at the students and smiled. Missy recognized her as the principal from one of the other schools.   Last year, her school and Dr. Dodge's school had gone on a field trip together in the Great Smoky Mountains National Park where they got a taste for how people in Cades Cove lived over a hundred and fifty years ago.

On that trip, they learned how horseshoes were forged, and how houses were built. They saw corn ground into cornmeal, and watched as a woman in pioneer dress turned sorghum into the heavy amber syrup that was usually served with hot biscuits on cold winter mornings.

"And   Captain   Cancer   Fighter,   Jordan Pickens."

Jordan was about Missy's age. He wore a bright white shirt with the words Captain Cancer Fighter airbrushed in purple along with an airbrushed purple ribbon, and camouflage pants and hat. He looked like he was already a private in the armed forces. He stood at attention, and saluted smartly.

"I'd like everyone to pay attention to what our guests are sharing with us this morning," Mrs. Mahoney said in a firm voice. When she spoke this way, everyone knew she wasn't kidding around. Causing a commotion, no matter how small, was going to be an instant trip to the principal's office.

Mrs. Mahoney stepped away from the microphone as Ms. Conerly stepped forward.

Missy liked Ms. Conerly instantly, mostly because she reminded her of her cousin Sammy's mom, Aunt Debbie.   She wore a long-sleeved purple shirt and black pants, which Missy thought looked very good on her.

"Hello students," Ms. Conerly greeted everyone.

"Good morning, Ms. Conerly," the student body replied in unison as they had done when addressed by Mrs. Mahoney.

"How many of you know about *Relay for Life*? Let's have a show of hands," Ms. Conerly began. A few hands shot up, but most students looked over at each other and shrugged their shoulders.

"A few of you. That's good. *Relay For Life* is an event that raises awareness of cancer. It also raises money for the American Cancer Society. How many people know someone affected by cancer?" she asked.

More hands shot up, but Missy suspected a few of her friends were reluctant to say if they knew someone who had either been diagnosed with cancer or had a family member struggling with it. This wasn't the sort of thing that most people talked openly about in her opinion.

"*Relay For Life* is a team fundraising event. When it comes to schools, we have *Relay Field Day* and *Relay Recess* for elementary and middle school students," Ms. Conerly stated in a clear voice. "I've spoken with your principal and with Dr. Dodge about having both schools help *Relay For Life* raise money to help us win the fight against cancer."

A ripple of enthusiasm rolled across the gym.

"Kids can make a difference just as much as adults. What we're asking you to do as a school is to get involved."

Missy sat up straight as she listened intently to Ms. Conerly speak.

"You'll learn how important it is to have good nutrition, and to stay away from tobacco and alcohol," she advised them. "You'll also learn about sun safety, and why regular physical activity is something you should make part of every day of your life."

To Missy, it sounded like the teachers were going to have lots of new stuff to add to health and physical education classes.

"Mrs. Mahoney and your teachers will share with you and your parents the ways that we hope you'll help us save lives," Ms. Conerly revealed before returning to her place in line. The students burst into applause for a second time.

Mrs. Mahoney returned to the microphone and quieted the students again.

"We'll be sending information home with each of you to share with your parents," Mrs. Mahoney advised everyone. "And now, I'd like you to welcome Mrs. Bowman and her son, Jordan."

The students applauded loudly to make sure Mrs. Bowman and Jordan knew they wanted to hear what they had to say. Missy was especially interested because she wondered if Jordan was training to be part of the military when he grew up just like she was training to be a private eye detective when she grew up.

CHAPTER 3

Mr. Jackson swept across the front of the stage and set a small box up in place by the microphone stand for Jordan to stand on. When he stood on it, he was the right height for speaking without having to stand on tiptoe.

Missy was impressed. Most kids never got to stand in front of an audience, never mind in front of an audience and behind a live microphone. Maybe someday she would get to speak in front of a lot of people, too. Trouble was, she wasn't sure she had anything important to say, and having something important to say was probably the number one reason a person got to speak to so many people all at one time.

"Hi, everybody. My name is Jordan and I'm Captain Cancer Fighter. I'm nine years old, and I've learned a lot about cancer in the last two years. I learned some stuff about cancer when my grandma got it, and I learned a lot more stuff about it when my mom got told she had it," Jordan shared bravely. "When my mom got cancer, I was sad and nervous. But my mom, she's a survivor."

Jordan's mom put her left hand on his right shoulder. Missy could tell she was proud of her son.

"My mission is to help find a cure for cancer. I want to raise awareness, and I want to raise money for research," he said in a loud, clear voice. He smiled broadly. "That's why I support *Relay For Life*, and *Relay Field Day*, and *Relay Recess*."

Missy looked around the gym and was happy to see nobody was goofing around. This was serious business. Everyone was paying attention to Jordan, and that meant everyone wanted to know all about *Relay For Life*, and *Relay Field Day*, and *Relay Recess*.

"Last year at the *Relay For Life* event, I got to wrestle a wrestler, and he was pretending to be cancer. I wrestled him down to the ground," Jordan said with conviction. "This year, I'm hoping everybody at your school and at my school are going to wrestle cancer so we can beat it."

Missy's brow furrowed. She wasn't sure how anyone could beat a disease just by wrestling it to the ground. Besides, she didn't think you could actually see cancer so how would you know when you should start wrestling with it? But there had to be a way otherwise Jordan wouldn't have done it, so Missy was excited to meet someone who not only knew how to do that, but had actually done it.

She waited to see if Jordan was going to go into more detail but he had already stepped down from the small box, and Mr. Jackson had whisked it away.

Mrs. Mahoney and Dr. Dodge stood side-by-side before the microphone. Each of them seemed to be bursting at the seams with a secret only they knew.

"Your teachers will explain *Relay Recess* to you when you go back to class," Mrs. Mahoney told the student body, "and then you'll have some class time to talk about ways you can get involved with *Relay For Life*."

Missy already had a couple of ideas in mind. The second idea relied heavily on getting her grandparents to agree to her first idea, but she was sure both ideas would be something her mom and grandparents would give her a thumbs up on. At least she hoped they would, otherwise she would have to come up with another first idea.

"Dr. Dodge and I have agreed to a wager," Mrs. Mahoney continued. Missy sat up straight, and eagerly waited to hear more about this wager. If the principals were going to bet on something, Missy just knew that *Relay For Life* was going to be as exciting as it was important. "Our schools are going to compete to see which one can raise the most money for *Relay For Life*."

The gymnasium broke out into enthusiastic cheers and whoops of laughter. Even the teachers were grinning.

"Let me assure you that this is all in good fun," Dr. Dodge added. "And who doesn't like having fun?"

The students loved the idea of the two schools competing against each other even without knowing what the wager was. It wasn't long before the student body became unruly, and it took two or three minutes for the teachers to quiet everyone down so both principals could announce to the students what the wager was.

"If Dr. Dodge's school raises more money than *our* school does, I'll be wearing *their* school colors for a week," Mrs. Mahoney revealed. A gasp went up from the crowd.

"And if your school raises more money than *my* school, I'll be wearing *your* school colors for a week," Dr. Dodge revealed.

Cheers erupted. Feet stomped. Loud whistles cut through the air. Visions of Jordan's principal rummaging through her wardrobe in search of fashionable clothes in their school colors danced in students' heads.

Missy vowed that she was going to do her part to raise as much money as she could to help her school win. She didn't want to see Mrs. Mahoney wearing the wrong colors. Mostly, however, she wanted to raise money to help save lives. After all, that's what *Relay For Life* was all about.

CHAPTER 4

Missy sat at her grandmother's kitchen table and slid a file folder across the table towards Grandma Barrett.

"I did lots and lots of research on the Internet," Missy said. Her brother Aaron had helped her find what she couldn't find on her own. Except for that, she had done the research. "These are the kind of invitations I want to send out to all your friends, Grandma. They're old-fashioned garden party invitations, and they have to have fancy writing on them."

Grandma Barrett flipped the file folder open and examined the first page. It was a traditional formal black-and-white invitation with a font that looked as if it had been scribed by a calligrapher during the Art Deco era of the 1920s.

"These are very fancy indeed," her grandma agreed, nodding her head. "Are you sure these are the kind of invitations we should send out?"

"Oh, I'm sure of it," Missy replied emphatically. "This is a very important garden party and I even have a special name for it."

"You do?"

"Yes, because very important garden parties have to have special names, so I already have a special name for this one," Missy assured her grandmother. "This is a *Pinwheels and Pearls* garden party."

"Oh my!" her grandma exclaimed. "That certainly does sound important."

"And it's important because the special name tells everybody that they have to come dressed up fancy," Missy explained. Her eyes twinkled as she imagined her grandmother's friends wearing their Sunday best, and being ushered into her grandparents' backyard by a butler. She wasn't sure where they could find a butler, but if they couldn't find one, Missy was certain that Aaron would be willing to dress up and pretend to be one.

"*Pinwheels and Pearls* certainly sounds like a dress-up affair to me," Grandma Barrett agreed. "I'm not sure I know what sort of refreshments we should serve."

"I know, Grandma," Missy giggled. "I did a whole lot of research. We should have cucumber sandwiches with the crusts cut off just like they have in the movies, and we should have pinwheel sandwiches. I already know how to make those because my mom makes them for me and Josh and Aaron for lunch sometimes."

"I'm sure your mother will be more than happy to help make pinwheel sandwiches since I'll be making cucumber sandwiches and hosting this fancy affair of yours," Grandma Barrett proposed.

"And tea," Missy added. "We have to have tea because that's what you have at garden parties."

"Not punch?"

"I guess we could have punch in case some of your friends don't like tea, but I think tea should be the drink of the day, don't you?" Missy asked.

"Perhaps we should have hot tea and iced tea, with some iced tea sweetened ..." She paused.

"And some tea that's not," Grandma Barrett said in unison with Missy.

"I think that would be fantastic! So what *kind* of tea do you have at a garden party, Grandma?" Missy wondered. Since she'd never been to a garden party, she wasn't sure what tea was the right tea for afternoon affairs in someone else's backyard.

"I would think that Earl Grey would be the way to go since we're having cucumber sandwiches," her grandma suggested.

"And pinwheel sandwiches," Missy interrupted. "Don't forget the pinwheel sandwiches. The tea has to go with the sandwiches or it won't work."

"Earl Grey goes with nearly every type of sandwich, Missy," her grandmother reassured her. "It's one of those stand-by teas that everyone knows, and if it's too strong, a nice dollop of honey or a bit of sugar will sweeten it up."

Missy smiled. "I even saw in the movies with garden parties in them that there was milk to put in the tea. That kind of mixed me up because I thought that was only for coffee but my mom said that sometimes people put milk in their tea."

"Your mother's right," Grandpa Barrett said as he strolled into the kitchen in search of his afternoon snack. Opening the refrigerator door, he rummaged about the top shelf before closing the door and moving on to the cupboard over the kitchen sink.

"James, what are you looking for?" Grandma Barrett asked, annoyed with Grandpa Barrett for clanking about in the kitchen.

"I'm looking for the mixed nuts we bought the other day," he said, winking at his granddaughter.

"Grandpa," Missy giggled, "when's the last time Grandma put mixed nuts in the fridge?" She liked watching her grandpa tease her grandma, mostly because it always ended up with Grandma Barrett laughing so hard that tears welled up in her eyes and rolled down her cheeks.

"I wasn't sure what I wanted when I was poking about in the fridge," Grandpa Barrett admitted. "The thing is I didn't see anything that struck my fancy in the fridge, and that's when I remembered your grandma and I bought mixed nuts the other day."

"James, if it's mixed nuts you're looking for, they're in the same cupboard they're always in," Grandma Barrett said, pointing towards the cupboard nearest the stove. "Just look in the pantry on the third shelf."

"Your grandma's got this house so organized a drill sergeant would be impressed," Grandpa Barrett told Missy. He winked an exaggerated wink at Grandma Barrett, and laughed.

"That's why I asked Grandma to help me with my *Pinwheels and Pearls* garden party," Missy informed her grandpa. "She knows everything about doing things right, and that's because she's superly organized everywhere all the time."

"Oh, I can think of a time or two when she wasn't so *superly organized* as you call it," Grandpa Barrett teased Grandma Barrett.

Grandma Barrett grinned as Grandpa Barrett made googly eyes at her. He followed that up with shrugging his shoulders at her, as if he was quietly sneaking towards Grandma Barrett even though his feet hadn't moved an inch. Then the giggling began. It wasn't long before Grandpa Barrett had Missy and her grandma in stitches.

CHAPTER 5

Missy knocked on her brother Josh's bedroom door. She knew he was in there even though the door was closed. She could hear his trademark machine-gun burst typing through the door.

"It's open," Josh hollered distractedly, leaving the impression he was in the middle of playing a video game online.

Missy turned the handle quietly so as not to disturb him, and slipped into his room. Just as she thought, he was playing one of his favorite games, and from what Missy could tell, he was at a critical point. One wrong word or distracting step, and he would probably lose his concentration, and that would probably cost him the level. It might even cost him the whole game.

Waiting patiently, Missy did a visual sweep of his room. As a future private eye detective, she never passed on a chance to hone her observation skills. Even if nothing in Josh's room had changed since the last time she was allowed in, that would be an important observation to make. But Josh being Josh, a lot had changed in his room. For one thing, he hadn't put his folded laundry away from the previous day, and it had toppled over on his dresser.

"Okay, Missy, so what's up?" Josh asked as he paused the game and pushed himself away from his computer desk.

Missy sat on Josh's bed and smiled. "I need your help with the fundraising I'm doing for *Relay For Life*."

"Really?" Josh replied, raising his eyebrows. Whenever Missy's sentence began with '*I need your help*' it almost always meant that someone was going to get talked into doing something they didn't know they were going to do.

"Well, I talked with grandma and grandpa about the first part of my fundraising idea," Missy shared enthusiastically, "but I didn't talk about the second part because they don't know how to draw like you do."

Josh grinned.

"All right. If it's drawing something, I can probably help," he declared. It was a tentative agreement that depended on how much work Missy's idea entailed.

"I need incentive. That's what mom calls it, right? Anyway, I need incentive so people will be interested in the third part of my idea," Missy continued explaining. "So I already talked with Roy on the phone and he said he could make the round circle things I need out of wood because he's really good at that."

Josh began to wonder where a garden party, wooden circles, and his artistic talents crossed paths in Missy's mind. Maybe she was going to ask him to sketch portraits at her *Pinwheels and Pearls* garden party, but that didn't explain why she needed Roy to cut out wooden circles unless they were frames for miniature portraits.

"The circles are going to be this big around," Missy said, holding her hands in front of her so they formed a circle. "That's a little bit smaller than my favorite apple."

Missy loved Granny Smith apples as much for their tartness as for the fact that they were smaller than most other apples. She liked to tell people that Granny Smith apples fit perfectly in little hands. What she didn't know was that her mother knew which stores sold the smaller ones, and those were the apples she bought for Missy.

"That's about three inches across," Josh told her, in case she needed to explain how big the circles were to anyone else. "But Missy, where do I ..."

"About three inches across," Missy continued, ignoring the fact that she had cut Josh off halfway through his question. "That's where you come in. The circles are actually happy sunshines except they have to be purple instead of yellow because *Relay For Life* has purple on their signs, not yellow."

"I'm not sure I'm following you. You want me to draw the purple sun for you to copy onto the wooden circles?" Josh guessed.

"Oh, thanks for saying you want to do this!" Missy gushed. She was so pleased her brother knew exactly what she was hoping would happen.

"Woah, woah, woah," Josh exclaimed, leaning back in his chair. "I think you jumped a few steps between telling me your idea and me agreeing to do some artwork for you."

Josh had already decided he would draw a purple sun for Missy, but he wanted to be asked properly and given the opportunity to consider his little sister's proposal. He didn't have the heart to turn her down, but he wanted her to understand that asking him to do her a favor wasn't always going to be granted just because they were brother and sister.

"Oh yeah, sorry about that," Missy giggled. "So what I thought you could do is agree to make the artwork of the purple sunshines for me. I don't have any money to give you but this is for a superly good cause. It's to help raise money for cancer research and important stuff like that."

Josh pretended to seriously consider the project. He hemmed and hawed, and watched Missy squirm in anticipation of winning him over with her eagerness to get started raising money.

"Please," Missy begged, defaulting to her best puppy dog eyes look. "You've been drawing since forever and I never saw something you made that I didn't love with all my heart."

Josh smiled. As a teenager, glowing reviews of his artwork wasn't something that happened as often as he would like. Even his art teacher at school didn't hand out compliments easily.

"I promise I don't want something really hard to draw," Missy argued her point further. "I was thinking a simple smiling face sunshine with happy eyes."

"Well, then, if that's all you're looking for, I think I can fit you into my busy schedule," Josh relented. "And you don't even have to pay me," he added, winking at his little sister.

"Oh good," Missy squealed as she reached into her back pocket and pulled out a folded piece of paper. She handed it to her brother, who unfolded it to see a sketch that approximated what Missy wanted.

"How about I come up with a couple designs of my own and show them to you tomorrow?" he asked. "That way you'll have two to choose from, and they'll both be variations on yours."

"I think that would be fantastic!" Missy agreed.

Jumping to her feet, she threw her arms around her brother's neck and hugged him tightly.

CHAPTER 6

Missy's oldest brother walked up the stairs to the second floor in the house, on his way to his bedroom. Missy came rushing out of Josh's bedroom and in her haste to get to her own room, she nearly ran straight into Aaron.

"Slow down there, Missy, or you'll knock yourself out," Aaron warned her. "Where are you off to in such a hurry?"

"I have to hurry back to my room and write down that Josh and Roy are making the purple sunshines for my fundraiser," Missy told him. "Then I have to figure out how to get you to do the *Pinwheels and Pearls* garden party with me."

Aaron was amazed at the amount of energy his little sister had. He sometimes got the idea that their mother had been like Missy when she was a little girl, but that was based entirely on stories Grandma and Grandpa Two Rivers had told them.

"Hang on a sec. I'm doing *what?*"

"I'm having a garden party and the whole neighborhood is coming! Maybe even the whole *city!* And I need you to help me with it or it won't work out. I don't want my garden party to be a humongous flop!"

"I thought all I was doing was helping you look up invitation ideas."

"That certainly helped," Missy said. "But I think there are other things you can do that would help me even more. After all, when you help me with this, you and me, we're *saving lives!*"

"You're aware I'm at college all day, every day, and when I'm not there, I'm here studying, right, Missy?"

"Sure, but we can work around that," Missy said. "Besides, you aren't always studying. Sometimes you're just goofing off and having fun. I know because sometimes I'm right here when you say you're goofing off so sometimes you're not studying."

Aaron hesitated. "How about we have milk and cookies in the kitchen while you tell me your idea?" Aaron suggested as he wandered towards his bedroom to drop off his knapsack.

"Oh, boy! A real planning meeting! This will be great!" Missy exclaimed. But then her eyes fell. "It's kind of close to supper. Mom might not like us having a snack even if we *are* having a real planning meeting. You know how she is about spoiled appetites," Missy warned Aaron.

Tossing his knapsack onto his bed, Aaron turned back to Missy and nodded. "You're probably right about the snack thing. How about we hang out on the back porch? That way we can talk and stay out of trouble at the same time."

Missy agreed. It wouldn't be as formal as a meeting in the kitchen, but the garden party wasn't going to plan itself so they had to get moving.

She hurried down the stairs, followed by Aaron who took his time. By the time Aaron reached the main floor, Missy was already at the back door waiting for him to catch up. Stopping by the refrigerator, Aaron grabbed two chilled fruit juice boxes before following Missy into the backyard.

Handing Missy one of the juice boxes, he asked, "So what's up?"

"I have an idea for making my *Pinwheels and Pearls* garden party even more superly special than it already is," Missy announced. "I was thinking maybe we could old-fashion it up and that way everybody is going to feel like they went back in time at least a hundred years to the olden times."

Aaron sipped on his juice, listening intently to Missy's plan.

"I was thinking that because it's a garden party and because it's in Grandma and Grandpa Barrett's backyard and because the invitations tell people to come dressed up fancy that maybe I should get a butler to do butlering things," Missy laid out for her brother.

"What kind of butlering things?"

"Opening the gate to the backyard to let the guests in, and making sure the punch is always cold because grandma said some of her friends like punch, not tea. And plus, she said we need iced tea on top of the hot tea," Missy told Aaron.

"I can probably help you out with the butler duties," Aaron assured his little sister.

"But you can't just do butler stuff and not have the right butler clothes," Missy advised her brother. "You don't need a top hat because that's part of what the men that were not butlers wore in the olden days. You have to have for sure a fancy jacket and a white shirt and white gloves so everybody gets that you're the butler."

"I'm not so sure I have any of that stuff aside from the white shirt," Aaron admitted, knowing that Missy would be disappointed to hear his wardrobe fell short of her wish list.

"How about asking your friend, Randy?" Missy suggested.

"Randy? You mean Living Statue Randy?" Aaron asked.

"Yeah, Living Statue Randy," Missy repeated, her eyes growing wide as another idea began to take shape. "And maybe your friend could come to the garden party and be the most awesomest living statue anybody ever in their whole entire life ever saw!"

"I don't know about that ..."

"He could help raise money for *Relay For Life*," Missy continued. "He could get dressed up like a pirate from the even more older old-fashioned days. Remember how he talked about doing that thing where if people put money in his treasure chest, he's like an animatronic robot and he tips his hat and he shakes the person's hand?"

Aaron considered Missy's idea. He had to admit she had a knack for creating fun events. From the time she was very little, she had always been interested in putting together all kinds of get-togethers to celebrate anything from a Welcome Home party after a trip to the hospital emergency room all the way up to a full-blown birthday celebration.

"I'll ask Randy if he's free that day, but that's the best I can do on that front," he told his sister. "I can't speak for other people's time."

"And what about the butler clothes?" Missy pressed her brother.

"I'll ask him if he's got anything I can borrow," Aaron told her. "We're about the same size so his stuff should fit me. But if he doesn't have anything ..."

"I'll go with you to the thrift shops until we find the right butler clothes," Missy interrupted. She didn't want Aaron to think she didn't appreciate his willingness to be her garden party butler. Besides, she was already coming up with a back-up plan in case Randy and the thrift shops didn't have the right clothes. Grandpa Barrett probably knew lots of people who had fancy old jackets and white gloves they'd be more than happy to loan Aaron for the day.

Missy sighed happily. This was going to be the greatest most fun-filled adventure-packed party yet.

CHAPTER 7

For as long as Missy could remember, her mother had held an account at the Tennessee State Bank, and Missy knew nearly everyone who worked at the branch her mother favored. It struck Missy as a place that might be interested in her second fundraiser.

The worst that could happen was that nobody needed her landscaping services, and the best that could happen was that more people than she could juggle would want to sign up. What Missy knew for sure was that if she didn't ask, she wouldn't know if anyone would want to know more about what she was doing.

"I'm really happy you had time to take me to mom's bank, Grandpa," Missy said to Grandpa Barrett.

"It's no bother really," he replied as he maneuvered his car into a spot on the far side of the bank parking lot. "I have some banking to do myself."

Missy waited for the car to come to a complete stop and for her grandfather to kill the engine before unbuckling her seatbelt. She did a quick check to make sure another car wasn't pulling into the spot beside her grandpa's car before opening the door and getting out. Reaching back into the car, she retrieved a file folder with all her fundraising information inside.

"Now remember Missy," her grandpa reminded her, "if the bank manager has her door closed or she's on the phone, we'll come back some other day."

"But Grandpa," Missy objected, "I can't let too many days go by otherwise I won't have enough days to do all the weeding people are going to have me doing."

Grandpa Barrett held his hand out to his granddaughter, and smiled. She took his hand gladly. As they made their way to the entrance, he added, "Your grandmother might have some banking to do tomorrow. Just so you know."

He held the door open for Missy and she scampered through to the next set of doors. She held one of *those* doors open for her grandpa, and said, "Ladies before gentlemen, and age … and age … and I forget the next part after age."

"Age before beauty," her grandfather told her. "Just don't tell your grandma I told you that, and don't repeat it to her either."

Missy nodded. She wasn't sure why she shouldn't repeat it but if her grandpa didn't think it was a good idea, then she trusted he knew what was best.

While Missy's grandfather stood at the table in the middle of the bank to sort his banking out, Missy confidently strode over to the branch manager's office. The door was open and the manager wasn't on the phone. Missy rapped lightly on the door.

"Hello, Missy," the manager greeted her, looking up from her paperwork. "How are you today?"

"I'm very fine, Ms. Loveday," Missy answered politely. "I know you're really busy because I see lots of stuff on your desk, but I was kind of wondering if you had some free time for me right now. I'm here on business."

Ms. Loveday grinned. "Come in and sit down, Missy. I'm never too busy to talk business with bank customers."

Missy sat in the chair closest the door, and gathered her thoughts.

"Have you ever heard of *Relay For Life*?" Missy asked. She thought it was best to find out right off the top if she was going to have to explain what *Relay For Life* was before explaining her fundraising idea.

"I do know about *Relay For Life*," Ms. Loveday assured Missy. "In fact, everyone at the bank knows about it."

"Well, I'm doing something special for *Relay For Life*. If you're going to do fundraising, the best way to make sure you get a lot of money for what you're doing is to ask everybody – friends, family, neighbors, everybody – to help," Missy began.

"That's what I've heard as well," Ms. Loveday confirmed as she folded her hands and listened carefully to what Missy had to say.

"My idea is a three-parter but the part I'm telling you is actually Part Number Three," Missy continued as she fiddled with the file folder she had brought with her. "Part Number Three is what I like to call *Quarter Corners*."

"I like the sound of that so far," Ms. Loveday said encouragingly.

"I'm offering to weed one square foot of garden for one dollar," Missy said. "That's why it's called *Quarter Corners* because a square has four corners, and every corner is a quarter and times four makes a dollar. So, you know, *Quarter Corners*. Get it?"

Ms. Loveday nodded. She *got it*, as Missy put it.

"I'm offering to do all the weeding for this branch as part of my fundraiser," Missy announced, cutting to the point of the meeting.

"Missy, I would love for you to do that but we have a landscaping company contracted to take care of everything," Ms. Loveday told Missy. "I'm afraid I can't help you out that way."

"How about this?" Missy asked, undeterred by the bad news that a landscaping company had beat her to the punch. "How about I put up a poster of my idea on the bank door and that way maybe some customers that need a good weeder person can have me come over and make my *Quarter Corners* a success!"

"As much as I would love to let you put up a poster, Missy, there are regulations the bank has to follow. Putting up a poster isn't allowed."

"Strike two," Missy announced, unfazed at having her second idea shot down. "I have another idea, and maybe this one is going to be okay."

"All right," Ms. Loveday said. "Fire away."

"I have these small posters I printed up on my mom's computer," Missy shared as she slipped one out of her file folder and handed it to the bank manager. "Maybe I could, you know, sneaky sneak give one to each teller. Maybe they can help me raise money by having me *Quarter Corners* their gardens."

Ms. Loveday read over the half-page handout before handing it back to Missy.

"If you could leave me with a few, I can put them in the staff break room," Ms. Loveday said with a smile. "That way if someone's interested, they'll know to call your mom and schedule a time when you can *Quarter Corners* their garden."

"That would be fantastic!" Missy squealed with delight. She counted out ten small posters and handed them to Ms. Loveday. "If you need more, just let my grandma know tomorrow. Grandpa says probably she's coming here tomorrow to do her own banking. My grandpa's here with me today, but tomorrow it's going to be my grandma."

"I'm sure these will do just fine," Ms. Loveday reassured Missy.

Getting up from the comfortable chair where she had been sitting, Missy extended her arm to shake hands as she had seen her mother do when saying goodbye to clients. "Thank you for your time."

"It was my pleasure," Ms. Loveday replied. "And Missy?"

"Yes?"

"You handled yourself very well," Ms. Loveday complimented her. "Very professionally."

"Thank you, Ms. Loveday" Missy giggled.

Missy left the bank manager's office satisfied that she had spent just enough time explaining her project but not too much so she was bothering her. It wasn't every day that someone her age had important business to do with a bank manager.

As Missy made her way to her grandfather standing at Ms. Cathy's teller counter, she waved at another teller she knew from other visits to the bank. Noelle acknowledged Missy with a nod. She was busy helping other customers and couldn't take time to do more than that, but Missy knew that if she could have, Noelle would have returned the gesture.

Three steps more, and she stood beside her Grandpa Barrett. She was certain he would be proud of how she had conducted herself. He would be pleased to learn she hadn't used up too much of Ms. Loveday's time either.

Looking down at his granddaughter, Grandpa Barrett asked, "Did you get all your business done?"

"I sure did," Missy confirmed. Peering over the counter, she revealed the nature of her meeting to Ms. Cathy. "There's going to be copies of my important poster in the break room for all the tellers to look at. Don't think you shouldn't be reading them because that's why they're there. The poster is all about my important *Relay For Life* fundraiser idea."

"I'll be sure to do that," Ms. Cathy replied as she handed Missy a fruit punch lollipop.

"Thanks," Missy said as she accepted the lollipop. "And thanks for looking at my poster. I'm hoping you have a garden at your house that needs lots of *Quarter Corners* weeding."

CHAPTER 8

Missy skipped along to her grandfather's car. The meeting with the bank manager had gone very well in her opinion, and she was looking forward to the next stop Grandpa Barrett had on his agenda. The second Missy and her grandpa were in the car and the key was in the ignition, Missy turned the radio on. She knew her grandpa liked keeping up on what was happening in the world, and the car clock was showing it was the top of the hour. It was time for a world update from the local radio station.

"You're listening to …" a voice jumped out of the speakers. Missy loved how the announcer made it sound like the best news and talk of East Tennessee came from the radio station where he was the announcer. Of course, the accompanying music made the news sound all the more exciting.

"Grandpa, what's cumulus mean?" Missy asked. It was a word the announcer used every time he let people know the news was on.

"It's a kind of cloud," Grandpa Barrett explained. "It's flat on the bottom and fluffy on top."

"Are those the ones that look like cotton?"

"Those are cumulus clouds," he confirmed as he turned onto the road on his way to their next destination.

Missy thought it was funny how her grandpa preferred driving along the tree-lined roads to get places while her grandma preferred the store-lined ones. The more she thought about it, the more she thought it probably had to do with the kinds of errands her grandma and grandpa ran. Grandma Barrett nearly always had the errands the required stopping at grocery and department stores. Grandpa Barrett nearly always had the errands the required going to places where something had to be deposited or dropped off, and that meant places like the bank and the Post Office.

As they drove along Ernest McMahan Road, she kept a keen eye out in case Marc Hightower and his biplane were high in the sky taking people on an escapade. Her adventure in the 1927 Waco Straight Wing a few months earlier was something Missy knew she would remember for as long as she lived. It had been one of the most exciting moments of her life!

"Grandpa, do you think lots and lots of people will want to sponsor my weeding fundraiser?" she asked. She wondered if her grandparents' friends already had people weeding their gardens for them. If they did, there wouldn't be any weeds for Missy to pull.

"If there's one thing I know, Missy," her grandfather shared, "it's that whether people have weeds in their gardens, most people are willing to do what they can to support good fundraisers. I think you'll do just fine."

"But what if nobody has any weeds?" Missy persisted. "What if they already have grandkids that come over on weekends to pull weeds for them?"

Missy's grandpa laughed heartily. Missy wasn't so sure she understood what was so funny about her question.

"Missy, pulling weeds is messy business and most kids aren't interested in working that hard to get dirty," he told his worried granddaughter. "Most parents have to squabble with most kids to get them to do stuff like that."

"They do?" Missy asked, surprised.

"Yes, Missy, they do."

"How come?"

"It's just the way it is," he replied. "Some need more convincing than others. It was like that when I was a kid, and it was like that when your dad was a kid."

"Except dad, he didn't have to get convinced when he was my age, right?" Missy wanted to know.

"Most times he was good at doing what he was told to do," her grandpa admitted, "but sometimes, he was short on motivation and needed to be told a couple times before he got moving."

Missy imagined her dad being her age and not wanting to weed the garden. She giggled. Sometimes it was hard imagining her mom and dad as nine year olds. It was a lot easier thinking they had always been grown-ups because she'd only ever known them as grown-ups.

"Did there used to be landscaping people back in the days when dad was little like me?" Missy asked. "Because if there weren't, then that's how come it was probably way easier to get kids to weed gardens back then."

"Missy, landscaping companies have been around for generations. Some places used to hire gardeners the way they hired cooks and nannies," Grandpa Barrett answered. "Kids have minds of their own. That's why it's important for parents and grandparents to make sure kids don't get themselves into trouble along the way. One of the best ways to make sure that doesn't happen is to make them mind their elders. Do you know what that means?"

"It means doing what you're supposed to do even if you don't get told and not be a jerk about it," Missy replied. She had heard her brothers use that term with each other from time to time.

Her grandfather put a hand to his mouth and coughed. She looked at her grandpa, concerned, but he appeared to be smiling behind his hand.

"Are you okay, Grandpa?"

"Yes Missy. It's just that you might want to reconsider how you said that last little bit," her grandpa suggested. "How about saying you should do what you're told to do without complaining?"

"But Josh and Aaron say ..."

"I'll be having a talk with Josh and Aaron about that, too, then," Grandpa Barrett interrupted Missy. "They know better than to talk like that, especially in front of kids your age."

Missy bit her bottom lip.   She hoped she hadn't gotten her brothers in trouble.   Glancing over at her grandpa, she noted his smile and crinkly eyes and figured that her grandpa would probably talk to Josh and Aaron in private and everything would work out fine.

The car came to a stop at the T-intersection before her grandfather turned right onto the street that would take them to Middle Creek Road.

"I hope that the money I raise for *Relay For Life* isn't too little," Missy said in a hushed tone. "I'm just a kid and I'm not going to raise thousands and thousands of dollars like grown-ups and companies do."

"Missy, it's not how much money you raise that makes the biggest difference," he said kindly. "What makes the difference is that you care enough to try to make a difference, even if that difference isn't thousands and thousands of dollars."

"Someday when I'm a grown-up and I have a private eye detective job, I'll get all the private eye detectives to do a fundraiser for *Relay For Life* with me every single year," Missy informed her grandfather. "Then we can raise lots of money to help people fight against cancer."

"Here's something to remember," her grandfather added. "When everyone pitches in and does a little bit of fundraising, they can fundraise thousands and thousands of dollars together. There's no fundraiser that's more important than another, Missy Barrett, and don't you forget that.

Every person who cares enough to help is doing their part in the fight against cancer, and that's what counts most."

Missy smiled.

CHAPTER 9

"We're here," Missy's grandpa announced cheerfully as he parked his car in the first open spot in front of Preferred Pharmacy. Missy giggled. When her grandpa made statements like that, it always sounded like they had been driving for hours to get where they were going.

Just as she had done at the bank, Missy checked for cars before opening the passenger door and stepping out. She closed the door firmly without slamming it shut. Slamming car doors was something her mother didn't like mostly because car doors didn't need to be slammed to be shut properly.

"Have you got your posters with you?" Grandpa Barrett asked Missy. Missy nodded as she waved a handful of small posters in the air.

"After you," Grandpa Barrett said as he held the door to the pharmacy open for Missy.

"Oh no, Grandpa," Missy replied. "After you."

"I insist, after you," Grandpa Barrett answered back.

"No, no, no, no" Missy chirped. "After you."

Missy had memorized the Chip and Dale cartoon chipmunk banter down to the last letter. It was an exchange she and her grandfather enjoyed, mostly because it was politely silly. It was a private joke between them that was very public in that every chance to kick off the Chip and Dale routine was started by her grandfather.

Not wanting to annoy customers inside, Missy slipped through the door and into the pharmacy followed by her grandfather.

Waiting in line were two elderly ladies who chatted about what was going on at The Island in Pigeon Forge, and a young woman with long dark hair holding a toddler in her arms. In the toddler's arms was a small stuffed animal that Missy thought was either a kitten or a skunk. It was hard to tell as the toy was black and white, and the toddler had it scrunched up tightly between the young woman's shoulder and the toddler's chubby arm.

It wasn't long before the seniors headed out the door with their purchases, with the young woman and the child following soon afterwards.

"Hello James," the man at the counter said.

"Hello Kelly," Missy's grandfather replied.

Turning to Missy, the man behind the counter added, "And hello to you, too, Missy."

"Hi, Mr. Snyder," Missy answered, smiling brightly at the pharmacist.

Missy always felt welcome whenever she visited the pharmacy. Everyone who worked there was happy and helpful, and no one ever seemed to be grouchy or in a bad mood. Even their shirts, which were a bright purple with white writing over their hearts, felt happy to Missy. By that, she meant that the shirts were bright, and they seemed to make the pharmacy even more cheerful and friendly than it already was.

"I know your grandpa's here to pick up something, but you and your mom were in just last week so I know you still have vitamins at home," the pharmacist said. His eyes twinkled as he spoke, as if he already had an inkling why Missy was there with her grandpa.

"We have lots of free vitamins in the bottle still," Missy assured him. "I asked grandpa if I could come along because I wanted to ask you some very important questions."

The pharmacist grinned.

"Now, if you can't do this, it's okay because I already was at the bank and I found out from Ms. Loveday that my first two ideas couldn't happen, but my third idea was a good one. I already know my first idea isn't going to work because you don't have any flower gardens in front of your store," Missy began, working up to the idea she thought might work best at this location.

Missy placed the small posters she had with her on the counter for the pharmacist to see. "Mr. Snyder, I'm doing some important fundraising to help save lives, and the money is going to *Relay For Life*. You know about *Relay For Life*, right?"

"Absolutely," the pharmacist replied. "In fact, we support important charities and events like that in the community all the time. When we fill people's prescriptions and explain to them how to live healthier lives, we're helping to save lives in our own way."

"And plus you give vitamins to moms and dads with kids my age," Missy added.

The first time Missy's mom filled a prescription at Mr. Snyder's pharmacy, he offered her a free bottle of multi-vitamins for Missy. Missy's mom thanked him for the kind offer, saying it wasn't necessary. It wasn't necessary, but Mr. Snyder explained that his pharmacy gave away monthly supplies of multi-vitamins to kids. He also suggested that Missy's mom run the idea of Missy taking vitamins past the pediatrician. Missy's mom thought it over a minute, and then graciously accept the gift.

"We absolutely do," Mr. Snyder confirmed with a big grin. "And since health is what we're all about, we're always happy to get on board with an organization that wants to save lives. So, what's your idea?"

"Well, I have two fundraisers but this is the fundraiser I want to tell you about," Missy began to explain in her official voice. "This one is called *Quarter Corners*, and for one dollar, I'll weed one square foot of garden. If someone pays me to come and weed one square foot of garden times five, meaning five feet of garden but only one foot wide, then they'll get a beautiful purple sunshine wood medallion to hang on their front porch. That's so people driving by will know that they're supporting my fundraiser for *Relay For Life*, and that we're fighting against cancer."

"That sounds like an excellent fundraiser, especially for a kid your age," the pharmacist commented.

"So I was kind of wondering if you could maybe put a couple of my posters up for people to read when they come to your pharmacy," Missy said, hoping the answer would be yes. "That way they'll know all about my fundraiser and they could write down the phone number I put on the poster and then they can phone my mom to book their space in my *Quarter Corners* weeding schedule."

Missy's grandpa proudly listened to Missy's convincing pitch to the pharmacist. He was impressed with how well she presented the idea.

"I'll tell you what I'll do for you, Missy," Kelly said. "I'll put a poster up by the door, and I'll keep one right here by the cash register. When someone shows interest in your fundraiser, I'll jot the contact information from the poster on the back of one of my business cards so that way they'll know how to reach your mom. How does that sound?"

Missy clapped her hands excitedly. "And that way they'll even remember exactly where they read all about my fundraiser so that's even a better idea than my idea all by itself," she added.

"That they will," Mr. Snyder agreed.

"And plus, do you want to know what my other fundraiser is?" Missy asked.

"Sure! What's your other fundraiser?"

"It's called the *Pinwheels and Pearls* garden party and it's going to be in my Grandma and

Grandpa Barrett's backyard, and people will pay one dollar for my brother Aaron to let them pass through the gate." Missy's voice grew a bit louder as she spoke. "And my grandma sent out these fancy invitations to all their friends, and it's going to be an old time-y garden party just like almost a hundred years ago. It's got an Art Deco theme because I love that kind of stuff. Want to know how I know about Art Deco?"

"Sure! How do you know about Art Deco?"

"Because that's the decorating style my Grandma Barrett loves the most and she has that decorating style all over her house," Missy explained. By now, her hands were gesturing wildly to show that the decorating style was all over her grandparents' house. "And sometimes when we watch black-and-white movies from the olden days, I see things in the movies that's like what's in my grandma and grandpa's house. Did you ever get to see their house, Mr. Snyder?"

"I can't say that I have," Kelly chuckled, "but from the sounds of things, maybe I should."

"Well, Kelly, you and your wife are more than welcome to come to Missy's garden party," Grandpa Barrett cut in.

"It's for a superly good cause," Missy added. "If you want to come, I'll ask my grandma to send you a proper invitation because in the old-fashioned days, if you got invited to a party, you had to bring the invitation with you so the butler would know to let you in. My brother Aaron's doing all the butlering at the party so that's how he would know who to let in. And plus, it's only one dollar a person to get in, and that's not so much money to pay to get in, right?"

"It sounds like a pretty good deal," Mr. Snyder agreed.

"So then we'll see you there," Missy giggled. "Don't worry about bringing anything because this is a garden party like from way long ago. That means we're having cucumber sandwiches and pinwheel sandwiches and tea to drink."

Grandpa Barrett placed his hand on his granddaughter's shoulder to let her know it was time to leave.

"It was good seeing you again, James," Kelly said to Missy's grandfather.

"Grandpa, wait!" Missy interrupted.

"Yes?"

"You almost forgot to get what Grandma sent you here to pick up. Remember?"

"I don't know what I'd do if you weren't my travel companion today," her grandpa laughed.

"That's okay, Grandpa," Missy replied. "You're helping me and I'm helping you, and that's what people should do for each other."

Grandpa Barrett pulled his wallet out and waited for the pharmacist to return with the package for Grandma Barrett.

CHAPTER 10

Supper smelled delicious, and Missy could hardly wait for the supper bell to ring. Unlike most homes where ringing the supper bell was a figure of speech, the Barrett household actually had a cast iron bell that hung on the kitchen wall. When supper was on the table, Missy's job was to grab the chain and clang the bell until everyone gathered in the kitchen.

The bell had begun as a joke. Having watched one too many cowboy movies months earlier, Missy suggested that perhaps her mother might want to buy a triangle the cooks used in the movies to call the cowboys to supper. Her mother said that she wasn't about to have her kitchen turned into a makeshift chuck wagon, and that she'd rather hear the sounds of a bell over the racket of a triangle.

Missy had repeated this to her mother's friend Roy on his next visit, and the visit after that, he brought with him a cast iron bell that he promptly installed in the eating area. From that point on, it was Missy's job to ring the bell for supper.

"Mom, are we having salad with supper tonight?" Missy asked.

Her mother often asked her to help out in the kitchen, and Missy liked to help because she considered cooking and baking skills worth knowing. They might come in handy should she find herself doing undercover private eye detective work in someone else's kitchen at a restaurant or in a billionaire's mansion. If she was doing things that a chef or a baker did, people might think she was a chef or a baker, and not a private eye detective.

But she also hoped they were having salad because ripping lettuce leaves up was always a lot of fun. Besides, it gave her some mom-and-daughter time to talk about important things like what she had overheard at the pharmacy.

Jenna Barrett smiled at her daughter. "Yes, we're having salad tonight. Maybe you could ..."

"Already on it, mom," Missy cut her off as she pulled open the refrigerator door and took out the head of lettuce in the crisper drawer. Settling in at the counter beside her mother, Missy grabbed the wooden salad bowl and began her kitchen chore with great abandon.

"So, how was your afternoon with grandpa?" her mother asked.

"It was superly great, and I got to talk to lots of people about my garden party fundraiser," Missy replied.

"That's good. I hope your grandma gets a lot of RSVPs so your party's a success."

"She says she probably will," Missy assured her mother. "And plus, grandpa has a couple more people for grandma to add to her list of people she's inviting to my party."

Missy's mom nodded her head as she stirred the tomato soup on the stove.

"When we were at the pharmacy, there were these two seniors there and they were talking about The Island," Missy said, delighted that she had so much news to share with her mother. "I love The Island. I love it so much I hope that on the next Girls' Day Out with Grandma Barrett that she picks that place to go to especially since it's her turn to pick the spot we're going to."

Walking across the bridge from the parking lot into The Island was magical for Missy. It didn't matter what time of year it was, just going to The Island meant she could create all sorts of adventures in her mind and act them out in this world inside a world.

Sometimes she got to ride the flying horse carousel where she would pretend she was either a fairy tale princess taking in the beauty of her father's kingdom, or a trick rider in the Buffalo Bill Cody Wild West Show except she wasn't doing any tricks because the show was parading through town on its way to set up show tents just outside of town. Sometimes she was just a kid riding a horse somewhere although she didn't always know where that somewhere was.

If she was particularly lucky, sometimes she got to ride The Island Express train, and when she got to ride The Island Express train, Missy always pretended it was the Wild West days and she was seeing the countryside for the first time. She especially loved waving at people who worked at The Island, and they always waved back at her.

On days when Missy and her mother were at The Island together, they would watch the artist at the Cosmic Pen draw live digital caricatures of people and pets. If no one was having their picture done, Missy and her mother spent time looking at the celebrity caricatures hanging in the windows.

"I was talking with your grandma on the phone while you were gone," Missy's mom said. "I can't say for sure, but I think there's something she wants to do at The Island tomorrow. Just remember to let your grandma choose the place she wants to go. No hints about where *you* want to go, okay?"

Missy knew exactly what her mom meant and she wasn't going to do anything to make her grandma change her mind about where she wanted to spend Girls' Day Out. Missy also didn't want her mom to think she had raised a rude daughter so Missy vowed to herself not to say or do anything that would make her grandma change her mind if they weren't going to The Island on their special outing.

"Anyway, when I was at the pharmacy with Grandpa, there were these two ladies and they were talking about The Island," Missy said, picking up the conversation where she had left off. "They were talking about *Relay For Life* and The Island. That was kind of neat because I'm doing something for *Relay For Life*, too."

"It's not polite to eavesdrop on people," Missy's mother reminded her.

"I wasn't eavesdropping, mom," Missy defended herself. "They were talking like we're talking right now. They were talking in regular people talking voices so I couldn't help hearing what they said."

Missy's mother chuckled.

"So anyway, they were talking about how The Island was giving a basket to a raffle that's raising money for *Relay For Life*, and you should've heard what's in that basket," Missy gushed. "It's so great I want to buy a ticket so maybe we can win that basket."

"So what did they say was in it?" Missy's mother asked, as much interested in the answer as she enjoyed hearing her daughter excited to share what she knew.

"Well, the one lady said that The Island collected lots of nice items from different stores. Things from places like that trading company place you like so much."

"Earthbound Trading?"

"Yeah, that place. And stuff from that place that makes the bath stuff like soaps and fizzies and that."

"Nourish Natural."

"Yeah, that place. Oh, and little hot sauces from the Pepper Palace." Missy paused before adding, "We should go there and get some more hot sauce for Grandpa. I think he's almost out of his favorite kind mostly because he told Grandma that it's chili making time again and he wasn't sure he had all the right ingredients for making his five-alarm chili."

"I'm sure he has all the ingredients," Missy's mother assured her. "Whenever your grandpa says he doesn't think he has all the right ingredients, it's his way of warning your grandma that he's going to be making his five-alarm chili."

"Is that because Grandma doesn't like really spicy stuff?"

"It's because your Grandma likes her chili to be closer to two-alarm than your grandpa's five-alarm version ever gets."

"Grandpa says it's because she doesn't want her curls to go straight, but I don't get that because you eat chili.   You don't use it for shampoo," Missy reasoned.

"It's just your grandpa being silly," Missy's mother explained. "You know how when I put the kettle on the stove for hot water it whistles when the water's boiling, and that's because of the steam?" Missy nodded her head. "Steam has a way of straightening everything out."

Missy giggled. She imagined her Grandma Barrett tasting the chili and her eyes growing wide with surprise at how spicy it was.   Then she imagined the temperature rising and her grandma's skin getting redder and redder until suddenly, streams of steam began coming out of her curls to the point where they straightened right out.

"So what else is in this basket?"

"Food and cooking supplies from Paula Deen's Family Kitchen, and a gift card from Timberwood Grill. Oh, and Arcade City passes and Escape Game passes, and if we won that basket Josh and Aaron would really be excited because they love the Arcade and the Escape Game place."

"That certainly does sound like a wonderful gift basket to auction off," Missy's mother said as she removed the pot of soup from the burner.

"I think we need to buy a ticket for sure," Missy insisted.

"I think we'll see about buying a ticket," Missy's mother corrected her, and Missy smiled. She knew her mother was going to buy a ticket for sure. It was too perfect a basket, and too important a cause, for her not to buy a ticket.

CHAPTER 11

Missy loved visiting The Island in Pigeon Forge, so when Grandma Barrett suggested that Girls' Day Out be spent wandering in and out of the shops and attractions, it didn't take too much convincing to get Missy onboard with the idea. Missy hoped she would get to ride the Great Smoky Mountain Ferris wheel. No matter how far away a person might be from The Island, the Ferris wheel was something that could be seen from a great distance. To Missy, it seemed like it was taller than any building she ever remembered seeing, even in the big cities she had visited.

"I have to stop in at the Emery Five and Dime," Grandma Barrett said cheerfully. "There's something special I want to pick up for this garden party you're holding in my backyard."

"That's great," Missy's mom piped up. "I want to peek at a few things in there myself."

"You go right along then," Grandma Barrett encouraged Missy's mom, "and Missy and I, we'll head off together to track down what I'm hoping to find."

"I'll find you guys as soon as I'm done then," Missy's mom promised before disappearing through the front doors.

The Emery Five and Dime was one of Missy's favorite stores, mostly because wandering the aisles meant she could pretend she had gone back in time to when the store was brand new. It had the same old time feeling she got from seeing '34 Ford cars, and so Missy imagined the store probably got its start about the same time as Ford cars got popular.

The store, with its cherry yellow and red gas vintage pumps and antique red and white soda pop machine in the store windows, always beckoned to her.

"I can hardly wait to see what your something special is that you're picking up," Missy said excitedly.

"I think you'll love it," Grandma Barrett said as she held the door open for Missy.

Just inside were two wooden candy counters with candies displayed in bins with glass in the doors to let customers see what was in each one. Longtime favorite candies like Turkish taffy, liquid honey drops, and kettle popcorn were neatly arranged along the countertop. Hard candies in butterscotch, root beer, and cinnamon flavors from a company that had been around since 1893 caught Missy's eye. She wondered what it must have been like back in the olden days to go to the store with a penny for candy and leave with a small paper bag full of treats.

"Let's see what's over in this direction," Grandma Barrett suggested.

At the back of the store, Missy and her grandmother found a new display. This one advertised embroidered cotton bags as well as sheer bags, and suggested pairing them with French soaps from the case. The soaps smelled wonderful, and reminded Missy of the soaps her Grandma Two Rivers made at home.

Not too far from the soaps and bags, Missy found note pads, and since she always had note pads with her to write things down, she wondered if she should draw her grandmother's attention to them. She found one with the letter M on a paisley cover but decided to save some money up to buy her own note pad instead of asking her grandmother to get her one. Even if she didn't ask, she knew that just pointing them out to her would mean her grandmother was sure to get one for her, and that wasn't really the point of Girls' Day Out.

"Oh!" Grandma Barrett exclaimed, and Missy turned quickly to see if everything was all right. Her grandmother was standing in front of a very old refrigerator with a great many magnets on the enamel door.

"This must have been put here since the last time we were here," her grandmother told her. "When I was growing up, we had a fridge just like this one. It's been years since I've thought of that old fridge. When my father, your great-grandfather, bought this for your great-grandmother, it was state of the art."

Missy looked at the fridge and giggled. It didn't look state of the art to her but it was attractive.

"I believe I was about your age when we got this fridge," Grandma Barrett continued. "It replaced the fridge he got her in 1938 when they were first married. Same manufacturer, too. The original fridge was still in fine shape but over the years, your great-grandfather had moved up the ladder, so he bought the new fridge and gave the old fridge to his younger brother. He did that to help him out since he was looking for one. He had just married his high school sweetheart, and they had moved into a nice little place on the edge of town."

Missy smiled. She knew that moving up the ladder meant you were going places. That's what her Grandpa Barrett had told her when she asked what he meant by saying that she was moving up the ladder when she started grade school. Every time someone was moving up the ladder, it meant things were getting better for that person, so Missy was happy to hear the fridge story her grandma was telling.

"I'll bet that's just one more reason you love this store, right, Grandma?" Missy asked, convinced she already knew the answer to her question.

"That and all the other memories that are part of Emery's," her grandmother admitted with a pensive smile. "There's just so much about this store that warms my heart."

"Remember when I was really little and I said I wanted to grow up to be a private eye detective?" Missy inquired.   Grandma Barrett chuckled.

"How could I forget?"

"This is the store you got those glasses from for me," Missy said proudly, "and I still use them for detectiving."

Missy had always taken good care of whatever others had given her as gifts. She took special care of things that helped her learn the art of private eye detectiving.   That meant that her magnifying glass, clue hat and clue coat were among her prized possessions.

But the possession that stood out at the top of her list were the first private eye detective tools anyone ever gave her, and those were the private eye detective spy glasses her Grandma Barrett had bought for her when she was almost five years old. What made them spy glasses were the mirrors on the inside of the lenses that allowed her to see what was behind her without letting anyone know she could see all that.

"I'm pleased to see you still remember those glasses," her grandma began to say, but Missy interrupted her.

"I still use those glasses because they're perfect for superly sneaky private eye detective work," Missy explained.

"I believe your mother told me that just last week when you were spying on your cats," Grandma Barrett suddenly remembered. "In any case, yes, I bought those spy glasses for you here at Emery's.   It was something that Mr. Emery himself suggested would be perfect for a budding detective like yourself."

"He was right," Missy agreed, "and if I ever meet him in person, I'm going to thank him for making such an excellent suggestion. I just love those sneaky sunglasses."

CHAPTER 12

"Evelyn," a senior with a sunny disposition called out to Missy's grandmother. "I haven't seen you in ages. How are you?"

"Hello, Ron," Missy's grandma replied with a smile. When Missy's grandma smiled, her eyes smiled, too, and Missy hoped that one day, when she was a grandma, her eyes would do the same.

"What brings you in today?" her grandma's friend asked.

"I'm looking to pick up a Smoky Mountain-opoly game. I know you carry them, but shopping with my granddaughter means sometimes it takes a little longer than usual to get to where I'm going," Grandma Barrett shared. While it was true that Missy liked to stop and look at the merchandise on the shelves, she had learned to appreciate the beauty of window shopping from her mother and grandmother, so it wasn't something that had happened out of the blue.

"And is this your granddaughter?" the man asked. "She looks a lot like you."

Missy's grandmother blushed, but Missy was quick to accept the compliment. After all, if she looked like her grandma when she was nine, she probably was going to keep on looking a lot like her grandma as she grew older.

Turning to Missy, the man said, "Did you know that your Grandma Barrett's first job was working for my dad?"

"At this store?" Missy marveled. She hadn't thought of how old The Island was, and for a moment, she wondered how long The Island had been in Pigeon Forge.

"Not at this location," he laughed. "My dad hired her when she was a teenager. She was looking for a part-time job, so we hired her."

"How long ago was that, Grandma?" Missy asked politely.

"Oh, that would have been in '57," her grandma told her.

"Back when girls went on dates with boys that bought them chocolate malts that had two straws but only one glass, right, Grandma?" Missy verified, certain she was remembering some stories her Grandpa Barrett had told her about the days when he was as old as her big brother Aaron was now.

"Oh, Missy, you have such an imagination!" her grandmother laughed.

"Was my grandma a good worker when she was a teenager?" Missy wanted to know. "And what kind of things did she do? Was she in charge of making malts and stuff like that?"

"She was one of our best workers," Mr. Emery told her, "and that's one of the reasons we put her to work at the candy counter."

"What was another reason?" Missy asked, excited to hear all about what her grandma was like as a teenager.

"Well, we always had the prettiest girls at the candy counter so your grandma was a shoe in," Mr. Emery said, winking at Missy.

"I remember the wonderful, delicious smell of fresh roasted peanuts," Grandma Barrett mused. Her eyes had a faraway look in them. "The fresh roasted peanuts, and the fresh chocolate ordered by the pound."

Chocolate by the pound!

Missy imagined a big truck parking in front of the store and two tall delivery men getting out, and walking to the back of the vehicle as Mr. Emery's father came out to greet them.

"How many pounds do you want today, Mr. Emery?" Missy imagined one of the delivery men asking Mr. Emery's father.

She guessed that Mr. Emery would have put a foot back inside the store to ask Missy's grandmother, "How much do you think we'll need today, Evelyn?"

"We need three hundred and eighty eight pounds, Mr. Emery," her grandmother might have replied.

"Make it an even four hundred," Mr. Emery's father might have told the delivery men (mostly because Missy thought four hundred sounded like the right amount of chocolate a store like this would sell back when her grandmother was a teenager). "And whatever we don't sell today, you can take home for supper, Evelyn."

She wasn't sure that Mr. Emery's father would have told her grandmother she could take home all the chocolate that didn't sell on days she worked the candy counter, but it was fun pretending that her grandmother went back home after work, loaded down with a paper bag full of delicious chocolate.

Missy loved when any of her grandparents told her stories from their childhood and teen years. Now that Missy knew that her grandma worked at the Emery Five and Dime General Store when she was a teenager, Missy was going to ask her lots of questions about what it was like back then.

"Did great-grandpa know Mr. Emery's dad?" Missy wondered.

"Missy, everyone knew everyone back then," Grandma Barrett said. "The original store's the oldest family owned five and dime store in the South, and when they opened the store in Sevierville, it didn't take long for the Emery Five and Dime to be one of the most popular stores in the area."

"Is it maybe even the oldest five and dime store in the whole U.S. of A.?" Missy asked excitedly, not knowing when the store first opened.

"The first store opened in 1927, with a second store going in over on Court Street in 1928," Mr. Emery shared. "In fact, if you go over to Holston's on Dolly Parton Parkway, you can see a photograph of that store hanging on their wall." Missy made a mental note to ask her mother if they could have lunch at Holston's as part of Girls' Day Out.

"I went for a ride in Marc Hightower's 1927 Waco biplane," Missy announced, realizing that the first Emery Five and Dime had something in common with Sky High Air Tours – the year 1927. "I didn't even get scared because it was so much fun. Have you ever been in a plane, Mr. Emery?"

"I have."

"Was it exciting for you, too? It was really exciting when I went with my other grandpa. He's not the grandpa that's married to this grandma. He's married to my other grandma." Missy's words gushed out, with each sentence running into the next.

"Would you like to know something else you might find interesting?" Mr. Emery asked. Missy nodded her head. "I served in the military, and my father served in the military." Missy's eyes grew wide. "He was a B26 pilot in World War II."

"When I get home, I'm going to look up pictures of B26 airplanes," Missy decided on the spot. "Then I'm going to read all about them because I like the history of airplanes. I've been learning all about Amelia Earhart and Charles Lindbergh and you know who told me about Charles Lindbergh? Mr. Hightower did."

Mr. Emery chuckled. "Seems to me that you're going to do just fine at school with a mind like yours."

Missy grinned.

"When I grow up I'm going to be a private eye detective," she told Mr. Emery, "so it's important for me to know a lot about a lot of things. Know why? Because sometimes if you know lots of things that other people don't know, you can find clues, and clues are how private eye detectives figure things out."

Missy stopped long enough to take a breath, then continued.

"I almost forgot," she said unexpectedly.

"What did you almost forget?" Mr. Emery inquired.

"You said you served in the military," Missy said, "so the first important thing I want to say is thank you for your service and for making the world safe for kids like me."

"You're welcome, Missy."

"Also, what was it like to be in the military?"

"Missy," her grandmother admonished. "Don't be a pest."

"It's all right, Evelyn," Mr. Emery assured Missy's grandma. Turning back to Missy, he said, "I was in the Marine Corps in the infantry division. That was back in '69. I was sent to Vietnam and saw combat."

"Did you get any medals?"

"I was awarded the Purple Heart with wings," Mr. Emery replied. Missy's eyes teared up. In her heart, he was a hero, and here he was, being an everyday grandpa type who knew her

Grandma Barrett from back when Grandma Barrett was a teenager.

"Do you have a photograph of your grandma reading any books with you?" Mr. Emery asked. He liked encouraging parents and grandparents to read to their children and grandchildren, and he always suggested they take a picture of them reading books together.

"My grandma has a picture of her and me when I was really little and just learning how to read, Mr. Emery," Missy declared. "It's this book that's a copy of a book from 1910."

"It's Little Red Riding Hood," Missy's grandma inserted into the conversation. "Remember when my oldest grandson was born twenty years ago and I came in and bought books so I could start reading to him right away?"

Mr. Emery laughed heartily.

"Over the years, I've bought books from here for all three of my grandchildren, and James and I have read all of those books with them," Grandma Barrett shared.

"Wanna know the best part about them doing that?" Missy asked. Before anyone could answer, Missy added, "Grandma has pictures of her and grandpa reading to all of us, and plus, she had a picture of her grandma reading Little Red Riding Hood to her when she was little! So probably your grandpa said to my great-grandpa that he should take a picture of that to make a forever memory."

"I wouldn't be surprised if that's exactly how it happened," Mr. Emery agreed, as Grandma Barrett nodded her head to confirm his suspicions.

Missy's mother re-appeared from the far side of the store.

"Hi, Ron," her mother greeted the store owner warmly. "I see my daughter is keeping you entertained. I just hope she hasn't monopolized too much of your time."

"That reminds me, you came in here to pick up a Smoky Mountain-opoly game, right, Evelyn?"

"Oh my goodness! I almost forget we were having so much fun reminiscing," Grandma Barrett exclaimed.

Mr. Emery guided the group down the aisle, then over two more. As they walked, Grandma Barrett and Mr. Emery continued reminiscing about her days at the store on Court Street, as Missy and her mother followed close behind.

"So what's this garden party you mentioned where you need a Smoky Mountain-opoly game?" Mr. Emery queried.

"It's to add fun to Missy's fundraiser for *Relay For Life*."

"My Grandma and Grandpa Barrett gave me permission to have a *Pinwheels and Pearls* garden party in their backyard to raise money for *Relay For Life*," Missy piped up. "It's going to be a 1920s style garden party. If you want to come, I'll just ask my Grandma to send you an invitation. Besides, there's lots of 1920s stuff that keeps popping up for this party like Mr. Hightower's 1927 biplane and your 1927 Emery Five and Dime and stuff like that."

"I think I'd like to hear more about this party," Mr. Emery said.

CHAPTER 13

Missy ran to answer the front door. It was by chance she had been looking out her bedroom window when Roy's truck pulled into the driveway. She threw open the door before anyone could ring the doorbell.

"Hi, Roy!" Missy greeted him. In her opinion, Roy was as close to family as he could get even though they weren't related. He was older than her mother, but younger than her grandparents, and he was always interested in hearing the latest about Missy's adventures and escapades.

"Hello, Missy," Roy replied. "I thought I'd stop by the house to drop off those wood medallions you had me make for your fundraiser." He held a paper bag out for Missy to take from him.

Quickly, she took the bag, opened it, and peered in. Looking back up at Roy, she gushed, "They're perfect, Roy! Thanks so much."

Aaron wandered out of the kitchen on his way upstairs with a sandwich in one hand and a soda in the other. Roy waved hello.

"What's up, Roy?" Aaron asked, swallowing the bit of sandwich he was chewing.

"Not much," Roy answered. "How's college going?"

"Roy just brought over the wooden circles I need to make the purple sunshines for *Quarter Corners*," Missy informed her oldest brother. She drew one out of the bag and showed it to him. "See how nice and round they are? Perfect circles!"

"They don't look purple to me," Aaron told Missy.

"That's because they're not done yet," Missy countered. "I have to paint them red first."

"I thought you said these sunshine things were purple," Aaron said, confused. He was certain that Missy had a plan that included purple as well as a sun design, but the chance to tease his little sister was too much to pass up.

"They are purple sunshines but the sunshines have to have a background color, and that's going to be red because red and purple go together," Missy told him as she waved her hand with the wooden circle about in the air.

Just then, Missy's mom, Jenna, came down the stairs with an empty laundry basket tucked under her arm. She stopped on the landing, surprised to find a small gathering happening at her front door.

"And this red paint you're putting on these things," Aaron continued, "I'm assuming you already have that paint upstairs in your room ready to go, right?"

"Not exactly," Missy admitted. She had hoped to ask Wesley from across the street if he had some extra red paint lying around in his garage. A month earlier, he had painted the front door of his house a bright cherry red, and she was certain he hadn't used a whole gallon of paint on the door even if he painted both sides.

"Missy Barrett, I hope you aren't expecting me to buy red paint for you," her mother admonished her. "I've already got a fair bit invested in your fundraiser."

"I've got some red paint back at the shop," Roy offered. "Probably enough to do all those medallions in the bag, and maybe a few more. Extras, you know. Just in case you need to make a few more."

Missy clapped her hands. "That would be perfect. All I have to do is get the paint and then paint all of these outside." She turned towards her mother. "Don't worry, mom. I've got newspaper set aside to put on the sidewalk so I won't get red paint splattered around my project."

Roy grinned. He knew Jenna was pleased her daughter was working so hard to make her fundraiser a success. He also knew that Jenna didn't want her daughter taking it for granted that people would do things just because Missy asked.

"I was wondering when Marc was going to start flying around town dragging a banner behind his biplane to let people know about your project, Missy," Roy teased.

"I don't even have a banner," Missy confessed, looking down at her feet in disappointment. There was a hole in her marketing idea, as her mother sometimes said about some promotions.

"I believe your mom knows Jonathan," Roy said quickly.

"The guy from Sign Master?" Missy asked feeling hopeful about Roy's idea.

"Roy, don't get her started," Jenna warned her friend.

"Oh, she knows I'm just kidding around. Don't you, kiddo?" Roy replied. He winked at Missy, and Missy winked back.

She hoped he wasn't just kidding around as he had told her mother. It would be a great idea to have Marc Hightower fly around town in his 1927 Waco biplane with a banner flying behind announcing *Quarter Corners* was in full swing. Besides, she had seen some of the banners that came from Sign Master thanks to her mom's business, and she thought Jonathan the Sign Master guy made the best signs ever!

"I'm serious," Jenna continued. "If she starts bugging me to talk to Jonathan about making a banner for her, I'm going to send Missy down to your shop to paint those things you made for her."

"They're wooden circles, mom," Missy shared helpfully as she showed her mother the one she had been waving around minutes earlier.

"I know they're wooden circles."

Jenna stepped down the three steps to the main floor. Aaron took the opportunity to rush past Jenna, and up the stairs to his bedroom.

"By the way, mom," Missy decided to ask since Roy could help her plead her case if things didn't go as planned, "I was wondering if you could print the purple sunshines that Josh is making for me. I don't need too many. Just one for every wooden circle and there's only …"

"Ten," Roy inserted into the conversation.

"There's only ten wooden circles and the design isn't so big. You could probably print all of them on two pages," Missy explained. "Three pages tops."

Jenna paused for a moment, then answered, "I'll print the design for you in exchange for you folding and stuffing envelopes for me on Friday after school. Deal?"

"Deal!" Missy said. She gave her mom two thumbs up, and beamed at Roy. "And if I need more, I'll just do more folding and stuffing, okay?"

Before Jenna could respond, Missy ran up the stairs shouting Josh's name at the top of her lungs.

"Well, Jenna," Roy declared, "it looks like Missy's fundraiser is going to be a huge success."

"It can't help but be a success," Jenna laughed. "She's got everyone helping her. She's doing a lot to make this happen, and what she can't do on her own, she's roped the rest of us into doing for her."

Roy rubbed his hands together. "Well, then, I'd best get back to the shop and start making some more medallions for her. I'm guessing that first set isn't going to last as long as she thinks it will."

"Thanks for helping her out like this, Roy. I really appreciate it."

"No trouble at all," Roy replied. "After all, it's good for kids to learn early that many hands make light work."

"They do at that, don't they?" Jenna chortled.

CHAPTER 14

Pacing back and forth in her grandparents' backyard, Missy worried about how well the *Pinwheels and Pearls* garden party would be attended. Her grandmother assured her repeatedly that nearly twenty of her friends had replied to the RSVP on the invitation. Her grandfather confirmed that four of his friends had readily accepted the invitation to attend the fundraiser, and would most likely bring their wives with them. Her mother advised her that good deeds were their own reward regardless of how many people showed up.

Folding tables were arranged at key locations in the garden, covered with proper linens and set with ironed and folded cloth napkins and small china plates and tea cups. On a separate table under a large umbrella sat a glass punch bowl filled with homemade lemonade with large slices of lemon floating among the lightly-tinted pink ice cubes. Beside the punch bowl were two large pitchers of iced tea – one sweetened and the other unsweetened.

The pinwheel and the cucumber sandwiches would be set out once the first guests arrived. Until then, they were in the kitchen in the refrigerator for safe keeping from Grandpa Barrett's pilfering paws, which is what Grandma Barrett called them.

"Knock, knock!" a cheery voice rang out.

Looking up, Missy saw a familiar face and grinned. It was her brother's friend, Randy, and he was dressed as his character Captain Ahadanad Venture. In one hand he held a small treasure chest where people could toss in tips, and in the other he held the small stage he stood on when he worked as a living statue.

"Oh, boy!" Missy shouted. "Thanks for coming to the party."

"You're very welcome, Missy," Randy replied, and extended a hand to her in the jerky, robotic fashion of a statue that wanted to shake hands.

She shook his hand, and giggled.

Aaron followed next, dressed smartly in what appeared to be an authentic period outfit for a butler working for a prestigious family of means. Bringing up the rear was Josh who had decided to assist Aaron with his duties, wearing an equally impressive outfit as an assistant butler.

"You can thank Randy for helping us find these suits," Aaron said with a smile. Randy tipped his hat in her direction. "Without him, your butlers for today would be pretty sorry looking excuses for servants."

Missy applauded, and Randy bowed in grand fashion.

"This is going to be the absolute most best garden party fundraiser ever even if hardly anyone shows up," Missy declared. Her hopes buoyed. Surely with two butlers and one living statue, the garden party would be the talk of the town. It would definitely be something party-goers would remember for a very long time.

"Hold on so I can get the silver tray for accepting the invitations from the people who show up," Missy told her brothers. "Someone will have to accept the invitations. When I come back with the silver tray, you have to tell me who the gate butler is."

Missy ran inside the house to get the tray, leaving Randy, Aaron, and Josh to chuckle over Missy's enthusiasm.

"She's pretty excited about this," Randy said.

The first time he met Missy was months earlier, when Missy had convinced herself there was a mystery going on in her mother's backyard. When she had left for school that morning, the backyard had been the way it always was, but when she returned from school later that afternoon, she had wondered who had erected a statue in the backyard without her mother's knowledge. Using her private eye detective skills, she had taken meticulous notes and written down very specific observations before realizing the statue was breathing.

"You don't know the half of it," Aaron laughed. "She's a real jumping bean."

"That's what our other grandpa says about her," Josh interjected into the conversation, not wanting to be left out of the camaraderie. "Well, that and a few other things like a spark plug, a fireball, a real live wire ..."

"Chipper," Aaron added.

"Chirpy," Josh tacked on.

"Bubbly," Aaron countered.

"Animated."

"Little Missy Sunshine."

"Top shelf, as they say in the Thin Man movies," Josh threw in for good measure.

The trio looked at each other. None of the words used to describe Missy missed the mark.

The back door swung open and Missy arrived with two silver trays as well as a beautiful bamboo bread basket.

"Grandma says whoever collects the one dollar admission fee can use the bread basket for the money," Missy advised her brothers. Josh reached out and took hold of the basket.

"Isn't this the one she uses for special dinners? The one she says perfectly accentuates the table?" Josh asked. He knew it was, but he also knew that Missy fell into a fit of giggles whenever he used the same words their grandparents used to describe things or places.

This time the comedy was lost on Missy who was focused on creating the right atmosphere for the garden party.

"It sure is, so you better take superly great care of it while you're putting money in it or grandma's going to have a fit," Missy advised Josh in all seriousness. "And here is the silver tray for collecting the invitations ..."

"What's the other silver tray for?" Aaron asked, certain he already knew the answer to that question as well.

"This is for proper butlering," Missy announced, shocked her brothers didn't realize what she felt was obvious. "You put a couple small plates of sandwiches on the silver tray and walk around so people can help themselves instead of always having to go to the table where mom is putting them out. But if people want to go to the table, they can. The butlering just makes it so they don't have to keep interrupting conversations to go get another pinwheel or cucumber sandwich."

Aaron and Josh nodded at each other, the unspoken joke understood by everyone.

"And if the people give you a tip like a dollar or something like that, you don't get to keep that. Butlers in the olden days already got paid by the master of the house," Missy continued. "That's money that goes to *Relay For Life*. So don't get upset when you can't keep those tips. They're not yours."

"I already knew that," Aaron assured his little sister. "I was just making sure Josh did."

"As if," Josh joked back.

The back door swung open again. Grandpa Barrett ushered Marc Hightower into the backyard. As promised, Marc wore his leather jacket and knee-high leather boots as well as the silk scarf responsible for the trademark barnstormer look from the 1920s. In his right hand, he held his goggles and leather helmet.

"Thanks so much for showing up dressed up in your biplane clothes, Mr. Hightower," Missy squealed with delight.

"No problem," Marc said. "Glad to help out. Besides, who doesn't like going to parties?"

"Everybody loves parties!" Missy gushed.

"So what do you want me to do?" Marc asked.

"You know, talk in 1920s barnstormer language," Missy explained. "Use words like *gee whiz* and *gosh* and *swell* and stuff like that."

Marc smiled. "Should I keep an eye out for any *news hawks* that might be around? Just so you know if they are."

"*News hawks*?"

"Yeah, that's 1920s talk for reporters," Marc told Missy.

"Oh for sure you should tell me if there's a *news hawk* here," Missy said quickly. "Also you should let me know if there's any *trouble boys*."

Trouble boys was what the police called gangsters in old movies, so she was confident she was using the term the right way.

It was a given at this point that the garden party would be a rousing success, especially since she had asked her mother to take pictures and post them online so people late to the party would hurry up and arrive. With two butlers, a living statue, and a barnstormer already at the event, people seeing the pictures online wouldn't want to miss any more of the fun.

She could hardly wait until she could welcome the first attendees. If everything went according to plan, they would come dressed in fancy outfits, and the ladies would be wearing pearl necklaces and maybe even pearl earrings.

CHAPTER 15

Within the hour, Grandma and Grandpa Barrett's backyard was buzzing with more people than invitations Aaron had collected on the silver tray. When she checked the invitations, she saw her grandmother had added two words to her invitations without telling her. The three words – *and a guest* -- accounted for the discrepancy between the number of invitations on the tray and the number of guests in attendance.

This was quickly becoming the social affair of the season in Missy's opinion.

"Missy, I'd like to introduce you to my friend Emily Kile," Grandma Barrett announced as she walked up to her granddaughter. The friend was a lovely lady with beautifully styled snow white hair and kind eyes that sparkled.

"Pleased to meet you, Ms. Kile."

Missy curtsied. She had watched enough black-and-white movies to know that this was how people responded to introductions back in the olden days.

"That's our Missy," Grandma Barrett chuckled.

"She's charming. Absolutely charming."

Ms. Kile shook Missy's hand. Remembering what her mother taught her, Missy made sure she didn't deliver what her mother called a dead fish handshake. She also remembered not to squeeze Ms. Kile's hand too tightly because that was as rude as the dead fish handshake.

"And I'm pleased to meet you, Missy. Your grandma's told me a lot about you."

"I hope she told you mostly the good stuff because if she told you some of the not-so-good stuff, maybe you'll think I'm not a very good listener," Missy fretted. She thought about the times she'd gotten herself into predicaments where she should have known better than to do what she did, and cringed. She hoped that her past mistakes wouldn't be held against her.

"Missy, there's a special reason I wanted to introduce you to my friend," Grandma Barrett interjected. "You see, years ago, and long before you were born, Ms. Kile started the first *Relay For Life* in Sevier County."

Missy's eyes grew large. She hadn't thought about how *Relay For Life* began, and now she was meeting the person who started it in the town where Missy lived.

"*Relay For Life* was *your* idea?" Missy gasped in amazement.

Ms. Kile laughed. "It wasn't exactly my idea," she told Missy. "*Relay For Life* began back in 1985 when Gordon Klatt decided to walk around the track at Baker Stadium in Tacoma, Washington for twenty-four hours to raise money for the American Cancer Society."

Missy listened intently. Learning how *Relay For Life* came into being was fascinating.

"He was a surgeon, if I remember correctly, and on that night back in 1985, some of his friends donated money to his cause just so they could walk with him. Now, they could have walked with him for free anytime because Dr. Klatt loved running marathons, but this was different."

"How many people gave him money?"

"I can't say for sure because I wasn't there, but what I do know is that almost three hundred people came out to that first event," Emily replied. "With so many people showing up to support him, he got to thinking, and in no time, he had a team of people pulled together for the first twenty-four hour run against cancer. That's even what they called it. They called it *The City of Destiny Classic Twenty-Four Hour Run Against Cancer*."

Missy was mesmerized. "How much money did his friends donate when he was just walking around the track but not at the running one?"

"I know it was a very large sum," Emily assured Missy.

"He's a very good man," Missy said decisively. Unlike many of her classmates, she thought everyday heroes were far more interesting than celebrities.

"He was a very good man, and he helped a great many people," Grandma Barrett added. Grandma Barrett was pleased to see her granddaughter take such interest in what Ms. Kile had to share with her.

"When did you make *Relay For Life* come to Sevier County?" Missy asked.

"Back in '99 I gathered together a wonderful committee of people I knew and we hit the ground running ..."

"That's a figure of speech," Missy interrupted Ms. Kile. "I know you didn't really hit the ground running. You just mean that everybody on your committee worked really hard to make *Relay For Life* happen, right?"

"Exactly. Everyone pulled their weight. We went to clubs and organizations and did presentations that talked about *Relay For Life* ... what it was, and where the money raised went," Emily continued remembering those early days. "The *first Relay For Life* was held at Sevierville City Park."

The event was going to be at Patriot Park this year, but Missy could picture what it must have been like when the event was held at Sevierville City Park. She had been to that park often. She had even gone swimming at the park pool on hot summer days, sometimes with her brothers, and sometimes with her grandparents.

"This year it's going to be at Patriot Park again," Missy said. She wanted Ms. Kile to know that *Relay For Life* mattered to her as well. "And guess what? It's at nighttime. Was the first one at nighttime, too?"

"It was *all* night long," Ms. Kile said, stretching the word *all* out for Missy's benefit. "People brought their tents and camped out overnight, and there were lots of different teams. Every team had sponsors cheering them on. It was simply wonderful to see the community come together like that."

"I'll bet you guys raised a lot of money."

Missy was certain the amount had to be at least five thousand dollars. If her fundraisers were successful, she was probably going to raise about a hundred dollars thanks to all the help she had putting together the *Pinwheel and Pearls* garden party as well as *Quarter Corners*. Without help from everyone she talked to about her fundraisers, Missy figured her fundraisers would probably cost her money instead of making money.

"We certainly did raise a lot of money," Ms. Kile guaranteed Missy. "We raised over a hundred thousand dollars that year."

Missy nearly fell over. A hundred thousand dollars was more money than she could imagine. Missy didn't want to be rude and ask what that kind of money looked like, so she tried to figure it out on her own in her head. She knew from watching television that sometimes brand new very good cars cost twenty thousand dollars, so a hundred thousand dollars would buy five brand new very good cars. She whistled her best whistle to show Ms. Kile that she understood just how much money more than a hundred thousand dollars was. It was enough money to buy five brand new very good cars and still have money left over.

"We ran all kinds of fundraisers from cakewalks to carwashes," Ms. Kile told Missy proudly. "We had a silent auction with lovely items. There was a little something for everyone to bid on. We even had tie-dyed shirts for the teams that year. What a memory!"

Missy could see that Ms. Kile had a lot of fond memories about *Relay For Life*, and she hoped that her garden party would be added to Ms. Kile's memories collection.

"Amy Harper took over two years later, and *Relay For Life* has been happening in Sevier County every year since then," Ms. Kile shared. "These days Sophia Conerly's the go-to person for the event."

"I know who she is!" Missy squealed excitedly as she clapped her hands. "She came to our school when we had assembly in the gym. Want to know who else was at the assembly? Mrs. Mahoney, the principal, of course, because it's her school, and Dr. Dodge, who's the principal of a different school, and Ms. Conerly because assembly was all about *Relay For Life* and *Relay Recess*. And plus there was Captain Cancer Fighter and he's a kid my age, and his mom! But that's not where I heard about *Relay For Life* the first time. The first time was when my grandma and me were going to Cassie's shop to get our hair done together."

The words seemed to spill out endlessly with no sign of slowing.

"I saw all these signs all over the place and they had *Relay For Life* on them and there were designs on them that made me think of purple sunshines and that's part of *Quarter Corners*. Just wait until you hear how the purple sunshines are part of *Quarter Corners*, Ms. Kile.   You won't believe how perfect everything fits together!"

"You certainly are a little firecracker," Ms. Kile complimented her.

Missy liked being called a firecracker, and she thought it made her presentation sound like fireworks going off.   It also reminded her of all the names her Grandpa Two Rivers had for her. *Firecracker* was something he would have called her.

"I almost forgot to ask: How come you got involved with *Relay For Life* a long time ago?   Did someone you know have cancer?" Missy asked.

"As a matter of fact, I did know someone with cancer.   I'm a cancer survivor," Ms. Kile revealed.

Missy stopped short.   She hoped she hadn't asked a question she should have left unasked. She hadn't meant to upset Ms. Kile even if it was done by accident.

"Missy, there's nothing wrong with asking why someone gets involved with a cause," Ms. Kile said.   "Once I was in remission, I wanted to return the kindness people had shown me during my fight, and I thought the best way was to help others who were fighting against cancer the way I did.   I didn't have to know who I was helping.   I just needed to know that I was helping others."

"Captain Cancer Fighter's mom is a cancer survivor," Missy said, "so you helped her get better, and you helped Captain Cancer Fighter, too, by helping his mom get better."

"I'm glad to hear that, Missy."

"My fundraisers aren't going to make a hundred thousand dollars," Missy apologized.

She hoped she would have at least a hundred dollars to donate once all the money from her two fundraisers was counted, but she wasn't sure there would be. It depended on how many people needed to have their gardens weeded, and it depended on how many people had shown up at the garden party in her grandparents' backyard.

Ms. Kile patted Missy on the shoulder, and smiled at her the way Grandma Barrett often smiled at her. It made her feel a bit better.

"Missy, it isn't about how much money you bring in ..."

"Except that I want to help a lot of people," Missy whispered so no one else would overhear her comment and think she was stuck on herself.

"What matters is that you're doing your best, and through your efforts, you've made a lot of people aware of what we're doing to fight cancer and help deal with it. You're only nine years old and you've come up with two very nice ideas," Ms. Kile praised Missy. "Next year, if you decide to do another fundraiser ..."

"Oh, I plan on it!" Missy nodded her head, and hoped she didn't sound like she was agreeing to another fundraiser just so she would look good to Ms. Kile.

"Well then, next year when you do another fundraiser, people will remember these two from this year, and I'm certain everyone will be more than happy to get on board with whatever you come up with."

Missy sighed happily. When she grew up and became a grandmother herself, she hoped she would be as nice as her two grandmothers and Ms. Kile all rolled into one.

She paused a moment, then decided it was time to announce the *Quarter Corners* fundraiser. She hoped at least three or four of her grandparents' friends would sign up for her weeding services.

CHAPTER 16

Grandpa Barrett stood in the middle of his backyard and *harrumphed* loudly to get everyone's attention. It took more than one *harrumph* but in no time, everyone was quiet and waiting to see what was going to happen next.

"Evelyn and I would like to thank everyone for coming to Missy's *Pinwheels and Pearls* garden party in support *of Relay For Life*," Grandpa Barrett said in a loud, clear voice. "We appreciate your donations in support of this worthy cause. In fact, we appreciate your donations so much that I told Missy just before everyone arrived that whatever money came in today, I would match the amount dollar for dollar."

A round of applause broke out, and Missy's heart pounded wildly. She hadn't counted the money in the bread basket yet, but she was sure there had to be at least thirty dollars. When she tried to count everyone in attendance, she counted twenty-seven people (not including her grandparents, her mother, the pilot, the living statue, and the two butlers) but she thought she might have missed one or two people since counting moving people was a difficult chore at the best of times. With Grandpa Barrett matching the amount in the bread basket, she'd have over fifty dollars to turn in to *Relay For Life* in the official donation envelope everyone was to hand in at school.

"And now, I'd like to turn things over to our lovely granddaughter, Missy Barrett," Grandpa Barrett said once the applause died down. He stepped back and Missy stepped onto the spot where her grandfather had stood.

Missy was nervous about speaking in front of so many people. But then she remembered Captain Cancer Fighter speaking on stage at her school and how she had wished she could have the same opportunity someday. She had thought then that the only time she could speak in front of a lot of people would be if she had something important to say. Well, *now* she had something important to say. And there was no reason for her to be nervous, either. If Captain Cancer Fighter could speak to a lot of people on her school's stage, she could speak to a lot of people at her garden party in her grandma and grandpa's backyard.

"Like my grandpa said, I want to thank everybody for coming to my *Pinwheels and Pearls* garden party," Missy stated mimicking her grandfather. "Also I would like to thank some other superly important people who helped me make this party happen because I didn't do this all by myself."

She motioned towards her grandparents, her mother and her brothers.

"This is my mom and these are my brothers, Aaron and Josh. You already know my grandma and grandpa. But I still want to thank my grandma and grandpa for letting me use their backyard for this superly special event. Without them, this garden party wouldn't even be a garden party. I don't know what it would've been."

The crowd tittered.

"And I want to give a special thank you to my grandpa for making sure everything was okay with City Hall for me to have a party in the backyard," Missy said seriously. "If you don't make sure everything's A-OK with City Hall, you can get into a whole lot of trouble. I know because my mom's friend Roy is always talking about how people need permits to do things, and Roy wouldn't make that up."

Missy's grandmother felt a fit of giggles coming on, and lowered her head slightly. She hoped no one would notice her shoulders shrugging up and down as she hid her face.

"You probably thought my mom wasn't here because she wasn't socializing like my grandma. You didn't see her because she spent most of her time in the kitchen making sure there was a steady supply of sandwiches and beverages. That way, nobody had to wait for more food and drinks to get made. She was today's kitchen staff one hundred percent with no extra helpers."

A few ladies liked Missy's detailing of her mother's duties. They nodded their heads and whispered approvingly to each other. There was no higher endorsement of a job well-done than the stamp of approval from a child.

"And Aaron and Josh, well, they're not really butlers," Missy explained. "They look like butlers today because I asked them to do the butlering for this garden party, and they did the best butlering I could ever ask for, don't you think?"

A smattering of applause broke out. Aaron and Josh looked at each other, not certain if they should stay in character or if they should be themselves again. They opted to stay in character since Missy's garden party wasn't over yet.

"Anybody want to know how come my brothers look like butlers?" Missy asked. Without waiting, she came back with the answer. "Because Chris and Jennifer at Sweet Fanny Adams Theater helped them out with getting the right butler clothes. Want to know how that happened? It's because Randy King asked them if they could help my brothers out by lending them the right kind of clothes. So a big round of applause for everybody at Sweet Fanny Adams Theater for helping out like that."

Missy was pleased to share how everything came together so well, and she hoped if people liked the butlering suits, they would take the time to see a show at Sweet Fanny Adams Theater because the whole show was old-fashioned. She waited patiently for the clapping to stop.

"In case you don't know who Randy King is, he's Captain Ahadanad Venture, the living statue. I think we should give him a round of applause, too, because he entertained everybody and he didn't even ask for any money like you're supposed to pay someone that works for you that way."

The show of appreciation went on for a long time before dying back down. Missy was pleased everyone approved of Randy's outstanding performance. She knew she loved his living statue work but she wasn't sure if it was because she was a kid, or because she was a kid and he was excellent on top of that.

"Sometimes he works at The Island so you should take people there to see him perform there, too," Missy continued. "And you should think about maybe hiring him to do parties for your work places because for sure, everybody will love love love what he does. He's the best living statue I ever met!"

In character, Randy walked over to Missy in animatronic style, holding his treasure chest in front of him. He stopped when he got two feet in front of Missy, bent at the waist, and handed her the treasure chest. He motioned to her to lift the lid. When she did, she noticed the treasure chest was nearly overflowing with paper money.

"And thanks to everybody that gave Captain Ahadanad Venture money so they could shake hands with the living statue part of him," Missy gushed. "I didn't pay him, but you guys did."

Randy extended his hand to shake Missy's as he had done with every guest who made a donation to his treasure chest that afternoon. When her face was nearly nose-to-nose with his, he whispered hoarsely, "Missy, I'm donating the money in this treasure chest to your fundraiser."

Missy jumped! There was so much money in the treasure chest, and Randy was giving it *all* to *Relay For Life* to help people fight against cancer. In that moment, she forgot he was supposed to be a statue, and she kissed him on the cheek.

"Everybody, Randy just told me he's giving all the money you gave him to the *Pinwheels and Pearls* garden party *Relay For Life* fundraiser!"

The gathering erupted with gratitude at the unexpected contribution. Missy sensed Randy might be blushing under his statue make-up but she couldn't prove it. Still, she was sure he had to be.

Placing the treasure chest down at her feet, she cleared her throat to get everyone's attention. She had more to share.

"Of course, Marc Hightower also made this party way more fun by bringing 1927 with him by dressing up like a pilot from the olden days," Missy added. "In case you don't know, he has a 1927 Waco Straight Wing biplane you can take a ride in. I know because my other grandpa – my Grandpa Two Rivers -- he took me to the airport and we got to ride in Marc's biplane with him, and it was so much fun. If you didn't go up for a ride with Marc yet, you should talk to him about when he can take you because you're not going to believe how much fun it is! And plus it doesn't cost so much, so talk to him about when you can have an adventure with him."

Marc waved at the small crowd, and Missy imagined that's exactly what barnstormers back in the day probably did when they landed their planes in fields and jumped out to greet the people.

"And now, I want to share something extra special with everybody," Missy declared. "Today's party was just the first part of my three-parter fundraising campaign. There's more! Lots more! So much more that you will hardly even believe your ears when I let you guys in on my other fundraiser. And for sure, I think you're going to really like what you hear."

CHAPTER 17

The guests were surprised to hear that the garden party was just the beginning. Over the years, they had been regaled with tales of Missy's adventures. Most of them knew about Missy's make-believe world where she was on the lookout for her nemesis, the Sneaky Itch, and his sidekick, Floaty Penguin. They knew she had brought Floaty Penguin to justice, and that the Sneaky Itch continued to elude her even though she never spoke about her make-believe world anymore.

They all knew that Missy was a creative powerhouse in that she never ran short on ideas. While everyone had anticipated that the *Pinwheels and Pearls* garden party was going to be among Missy's best ideas, they hadn't anticipated that perhaps she would run with a companion idea to complement it.

"When you look around this backyard, what do you see?" Missy asked. She had watched her teacher do this often in class, and it always led to a lot of students throwing their hands up in the air in the hopes they would be called on to answer. She waited, but no one's hand went up.

"Flowers, right?" she tossed out, hinting that there were other correct answers. Still no one made a move to offer up any other answers.

Taking note that Missy was looking for someone to take up the slack, Marc made a suggestion. "Grass. Nicely manicured grass."

Missy was delighted that Marc had spoken up.

"Anything else?" she asked, hoping that others would toss out ideas.

"Trees," one guest answered.

"A very nice garden with beautiful tomato plants," another added.

"The best garden party I have ever attended," a big voice from behind the crowd boomed. Choruses of *hear, hear* could be heard among the attendees.

"And purple pinwheels planted in the flower beds because that's what I put there this morning when I got here with my mom to set up the party," Missy announced, pointing in the direction of pinwheels that twirled gently whenever there was a breeze.

"Now," Missy asked, building on the momentum, "what do you *not* see in this very same garden?"

"The police," Josh teased, and everyone burst out laughing.

Missy gave her brother a warning look. She didn't want her important announcement to get lost in the joking around. Besides, her grandpa had talked to City Hall and that was to make sure the police weren't going to show up and give people citations for being at a party the police didn't know about in the first place.

116

"No! Weeds. Weeds are what you don't see. The reason why you don't see weeds is because my grandma yanks them out every time she sees them growing in her garden," Missy pointed out. "Now, my grandma doesn't like getting dirty, so sometimes I get rid of those weeds for her, and she likes that a lot more than doing it herself. That's where the next part of my idea comes in."

Missy walked over to the umbrella-covered table, and reached for a file folder that lay against one of the table legs. Attached to the file was a pen neatly clipped to the cover.

"In this file are sign-up sheets," Missy began. "But before people get the wrong idea, I'm not asking people to sign up to get the weeds out of my grandma's backyard. This is a sign-up sheet for people that want me, Missy Barrett, to go to their house to yank weeds out of their own gardens."

A rumble of approval could be heard spreading across the yard.

"This part of the fundraiser is called *Quarter Corners* and that's because I'm only asking people to pay one whole dollar for every square foot of their yard they want weeds pulled out of," Missy continued, taking on a business-like approach to selling her idea. "It's called *Quarter Corners* because there's four quarters in every dollar. That's one quarter on every corner of a square."

"I'm only available for flower beds and gardens because that's what I'm best at when it comes to yanking weeds out one hundred percent,"

Missy advertised to the group. "But wait, that's not all."

Reaching into the pocket of her dress, she pulled out one of the wooden medallions with the purple sunshine she put together.

"When you pay for five squares at a time, you get this beautiful decoration to hang on your porch that lets people know that you donated to my *Relay For Life* fundraiser. The wood for these was generously donated and hand-carved by my friend Roy. I almost forgot to say thank you to him at this party until right now, so I'm sorry about that. But the good news is that you can see how beautiful his hard work is up close when you look at this perfectly round medallion."

Everyone applauded appreciatively.

"And for those of you who don't have gardens or flower beds, or you already have grandkids that help at your house, you can still get one of these beautiful decorative handmade commemorative medallions with a purple sunshine designed by my brother, Josh, by donating five dollars today."

Grandpa Barrett smiled broadly. Missy's presentation ranked near the top of the all-time best sales presentations he had ever heard.

"Also, if you don't have any bills on you, I'll take checks. My grandma and grandpa know all of you because that's how you got invited to this party, and that means your checks are good. I don't have a credit card machine so I can't take credit cards or debit cards. But I can take real money, and I can take checks."

Missy didn't want to lose any sponsors because they only had checks. She knew that as long as the checks were made out to the American Cancer Society, everything would be fine.

"So, who's going to be first in line to sign up for some *Quarter Corners*?" Missy asked, nodding her head as if it might sway some who were considering the proposition but hadn't quite made up their minds. "My work is guaranteed and plus, I have a lot of experience doing excellent weeding. Just look at my grandma and grandpa's backyard for proof!"

CHAPTER 18

The garden party guests were long gone as Missy sat at her grandparents' kitchen table. Grandma Barrett loaded up the dishwasher as Grandpa Barrett put the linens in the washing machine to wash. Josh and Aaron, who had changed out of their butlering suits into jeans and t-shirts after the party, wrestled the fold-up tables and chairs into the basement for storage until Roy could pick them up and return them to their rightful owners.

Missy and her mother carefully separated the money into four piles: One pile was garden party admissions paid upon entry. One pile was donations made to Captain Ahadanad Venture who then donated it to the garden party fundraiser. One pile was tips that were collected on the silver platter throughout the party. The last pile was money collected for *Quarter Corners*.

"So how did you do?" Grandpa Barrett asked, pulling out a chair and sitting down beside Missy.

"Remember when you said before the party that you would write a check that was equal with how much money got raised?" Missy reminded her grandfather. Josh and Aaron wandered into the kitchen, and sat on the stools by the counter.

Grandpa Barrett reached into his jacket pocket, pulled out his checkbook, and laid it on the table.

"How well did you do?" Grandma Barrett asked as she took a place next to Grandpa Barrett at the table. "Did you get thirty dollars?"

Missy giggled.

"Captain Ahadanad Venture got almost thirty dollars all by himself," Missy announced, pleased party-goers had enjoyed the living statue entertainment enough to throw so much money into his treasure chest. "Mom says that there were twenty-one invitations turned in but there was way more than twenty-one dollars in the bread basket at the gate. Mom says there was fifty-two dollars in the bread basket."

It was true that fifty-two dollars made it into the bread basket, but there hadn't been fifty-two guests at the party. Some of the guests had paid five dollars to get in instead of the one dollar that was being asked at the gate. Josh hadn't said a word about it, choosing to believe that the additional money was a donation to the cause which was exactly what the extra money was meant to be.

"I'll round up Captain Venture's to thirty dollars and add that to the fifty-two dollars from the gate," Grandpa Barrett said with a smile. "How much more did you get?"

"You won't believe how much silver tray money there was!" Missy gushed. She had truly been surprised when more than a few coins were tossed onto the tray. It got to a point where Aaron had to borrow the silver candy dish to place on the tray to keep the tips from falling off and getting lost in the grass.

"Ten dollars?" Grandma Barrett ventured a guess.

"More!"

"Fifteen?"

"More!"

"Well, it couldn't possibly be more than twenty dollars," Grandma Barrett said.

"Almost eighteen dollars, Grandma! Aaron got almost eighteen dollars, and he said that he would give me some money to make it twenty dollars even. Isn't that great?"

Grandpa Barrett pulled the pen from the checkbook sleeve. He had a sneaking suspicion that his offer to match whatever was raised was going to be slightly more than he had originally anticipated.

"But here's the best part," Missy said, excited by the event's success. "So many people talked to me about *Quarter Corners* that I'm going to be weeding gardens for at least one whole month and everybody paid me ahead of time. Isn't that great?"

"How many of those square feet did you agree to weed, Missy?" Grandpa Barrett asked cautiously.

"Forty-three!" Missy squealed, her eyes shining bright. "And you know what? I can weed four of those squares in one hour and that's doing a superly great job because that's how much excellent weeding I do when I'm here helping you guys out."

"She does do at least four squares in an hour," Grandma Barrett confirmed to Grandpa Barrett, "and she does an excellent job of getting every single weed."

"Missy could get eleven hours of weeding done in two weekends," Josh chortled. He already guessed that he would be asked to accompany her to allow Missy to complete her gardening agreements but he didn't mind. When he was Missy's age, Aaron had accompanied him on a few fundraising activities his Boy Scout troop had agreed to do.

"I'm thinking about people that maybe might have a certain weekend in mind so it fits in with their planting schedules and stuff like that," Missy announced.

She had considered the possibility that some people might want the weeding done just before they planted flowers and shrubs while others might want the weeding done two or three weeks after they planted flowers and shrubs.

Grandma Barrett laughed heartily. "Well, James, you did teach our granddaughter that some plants are started indoors earlier than others, and you did teach her that some plants are transplanted outdoors earlier than others. You can't blame her for being a conscientious gardener."

"I guess I can't, can I?" Grandpa Barrett grinned. "So that's forty-three dollars for *Quarter Corners* added to the total, right?"

Missy's mother chuckled. As with most of Missy's ideas, they never turned out as expected, and most of it had to do with Missy's enthusiasm for doing things as best she could.

"Grandpa, some of yours and Grandma's friends paid for squares they don't even have!" Missy exclaimed, slapping her hands down on the table as if she had just finished eating a hearty meal. "Guess how many extra squares got paid for that your friends don't have?"

Grandpa Barrett was almost afraid to ask except that he was also delighted to hear Missy's hard work had paid off handsomely. He held up his right hand as if to ask if five invisible squares had been added to the tally. Missy shook her head. He opened and closed his hand twice to indicate ten invisible squares, and again Missy shook her head.

"Twelve extra squares, Grandpa," Missy shared breathlessly. "Your friends paid for twelve extra squares they don't even have. How crazy great is that?"

"Pretty crazy great if you ask me," replied Grandma Barrett as she gently nudged Grandpa Barrett with her elbow.

"Who knew our friends had so many squares they don't have, and all of those imaginary squares need weeding?" Grandpa Barrett joked back.

"So that's thirty dollars from the living statue, fifty-two from the gate, twenty from the silver plate tips, forty-three for real squares, twelve for imaginary squares, and another three bucks from me to make it an even hundred and sixty dollars," Josh tallied loudly. "With your matching donation, Grandpa, that makes three hundred and twenty dollars Missy raised for *Relay For Life*."

Missy's family burst into a round of applause.

"Congratulations, Missy," her grandfather said proudly as he began writing out a check. "You did a great job, and I'll bet your school is going to raise the most money. Isn't it going to be fun seeing Dr. Dodge wearing your school colors for a whole week?"

"Actually, Grandpa," Missy admitted, "I'm way more excited that so many people are going to get help from all the money everyone at both schools are giving to *Relay For Life*. I really don't care who has to wear what colors as long as we're helping people that need help. And we're saving lives."

"Missy, I think I forgot to tell your Grandpa I was putting fifteen dollars in as well," Missy's mother interrupted.

"Oh, I already figured you had fifteen or so dollars to donate to the cause," Grandpa Barrett revealed. "That's why the check is for one hundred and seventy-five dollars."

He picked up the checkbook and showed it to Missy. Her eyes grew wide as she saw her grandfather had already allotted for the additional fifteen dollars from Missy's mother in writing his matching funds check.

"You guys are all the best," Missy said emotionally. "Thanks for helping me get so much money for *Relay For Life*. We did it together. That's what families do. They do important things together, and we're helping other families so they can do important things together, too."

Just then, the doorbell rang.

"Who can that be?" Grandma Barrett asked.

"Don't get up, Grandma. I'll go check," Aaron said.

Moments later, he reappeared.

"Who was it?" Grandpa Barrett asked.

"It was a delivery man," Aaron announced. "With something for Missy."

He handed an envelope to his little sister.

Missy couldn't imagine who would be sending her anything at her Grandma and Grandpa Barrett's house. She wasn't even sure who would know to send her anything at this address unless it was someone who had been at *the Pinwheels and Pearls* garden party.

Inside the envelope was a second envelope, which she tore open. Inside, Missy found a card and she opened it excitedly in anticipation of what might be inside.

Maybe it was a letter from Captain Cancer Fighter telling her he heard about her *Pinwheels and Pearls* garden party.

Maybe it was from her principal saying that so many kids had successful fundraisers that they were going to hire a security guard to collect and protect all the money until it could be delivered to Ms. Conerly.

As she pulled the card out of the envelope, a piece of paper fell out. Missy picked it up and put it down on the table for everyone to see. It was a personal check from Grandma and Grandpa Two Rivers, and made out to the American Cancer Society.

Across the front of the card was one word printed in large purple letters: **Congratulations!**

"It's from Grandpa Two Rivers!" Missy shouted excitedly. "I can tell from the printing!"

Missy looked directly at her Grandma Barrett. "They couldn't make it today so it's nice my other grandma and grandpa sent this note."

"I took a lot of photographs, Missy," Grandma Barrett said kindly. "When your Grandma Two Rivers phoned to say they had a prior engagement, I decided right then and there I'd have to send her photos of your garden party so they could see how successful it was."

"And so they could see how much fun it was, right?" Missy added.

"Thanks for doing that," Missy giggled, giving her grandma a quick hug. "You're the best!"

Missy opened the card and read the note aloud.

Dear Missy,

We're both sorry we were unable to make it for your Pinwheels and Pearls garden party fundraiser, but enclosed please find a check for twenty-five dollars made payable to the American Cancer Society. That's two dollars for the price of admission for the two of us, and twenty three just because.

We're proud of you for working so hard to help so many people!

Love,
Grandma and Grandpa Two Rivers

"Wow!" Josh said in a low voice. "Who knew that Grandma and Grandpa Two Rivers had twenty-three imaginary squares for Missy to weed."

"Who knew the party would raise two hundred dollars, and that Grandpa Barrett would write a check for another two hundred dollars," Missy burbled.

Grandpa Barrett smiled and resigned himself to tearing up the check he had just written. He was going to have to write a new check to include Grandma and Grandpa Two Rivers' contribution. After all, he *did* promise to match donations to Missy's fundraiser dollar-for-dollar, and that's exactly what he was going to do.

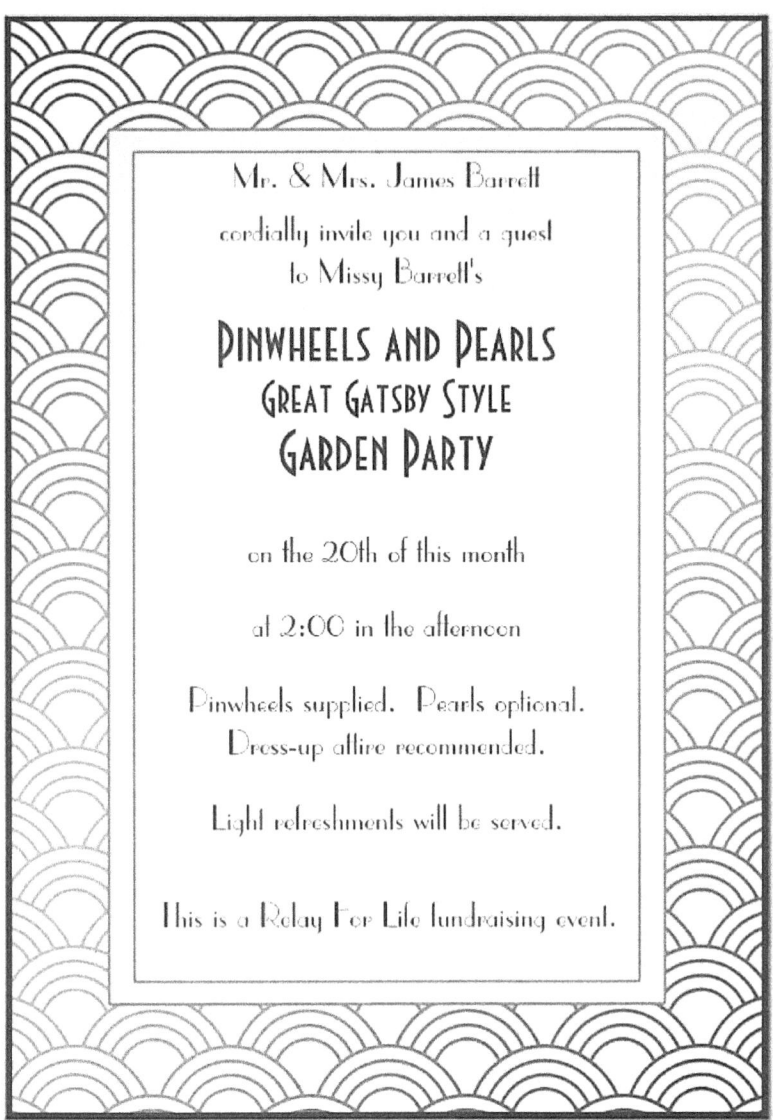

Mr. & Mrs. James Barrett

cordially invite you and a guest

to Missy Barrett's

PINWHEELS AND PEARLS
GREAT GATSBY STYLE
GARDEN PARTY

on the 20th of this month

at 2:00 in the afternoon

Pinwheels supplied. Pearls optional.
Dress-up attire recommended.

Light refreshments will be served.

This is a Relay For Life fundraising event.

BUSINESSES MENTIONED
IN THIS BOOK

ARCADE CITY
131 The Island Drive, Suite 1105, Pigeon Forge, TN
www.AmusementEntertainmentGroup.com

COSMIC PEN
131 The Island Drive, Suite 5102, Pigeon Forge, TN
www.cosmicpen.com

EMERY 5 & 10 GENERAL STORE
131 The Island Drive, Suite 5105, Pigeon Forge, TN
www.emery510.com

EARTHBOUND TRADING
131 The Island Drive, Suite 5116, Pigeon Forge, TN
www.earthboundtrading.com/

ESCAPE GAME
131 The Island Drive, Suite 9139, Pigeon Forge, TN
www.TheEscapeGamePigeonForge.com

THE ISLAND AT PIGEON FORGE
131 The Island Drive, Pigeon Forge, TN
www.IslandInPigeonForge.com

HOLSTEN'S
639 Dolly Parton Pkwy, Sevierville, TN
www.holstonskitchen.com/location/sevierville-tn

NOURISH NATURAL BATH PRODUCTS

131 The Island Drive, Suite 5115, Pigeon Forge, TN

www.nourishsavannah.com

PAULA DEEN'S FAMILY KITCHEN

131 The Island Drive, Suite 8101, Pigeon Forge, TN

www.PaulDeensFamilyKitchen.com

PEPPER PALACE

3275 Newport Highway S, Unit #5, Sevierville, TN

www.pepperpalace.com

PREFERRED PHARMACY

1024 Middle Creek Rd #1, Sevierville, TN

www.preferredpharmacyrx.com

RELAY FOR LIFE OF SEVIER COUNTY

www.facebook.com/1relayforlifeofseviercounty

SHEAR MADNESS BEAUTY AND BEYOND

212 Collier Drive, Sevierville, TN

www.shearmadnessbeauty.com

SIGN MASTER

110 Oak Cluster, Suite 1, Sevierville, TN

www.SignMasterTN.com

SKY HIGH AIR TOURS

134 Air Museum Way, Sevierville, TN

www.skyhighairtours.com

SWEET FANNY ADAMS THEATER
461 Parkway, Gatlinburg, TN
www.sweetfannyadams.com

TENNESSEE STATE BANK
1375 Dolly Parton Parkway, Sevierville, TN
www.tnstatebank.com

TIMBERWOOD GRILL
131 The Island Drive, Suite 1101, Pigeon Forge, TN
www.TimberwoodGrillPF.com

REAL PEOPLE
IN THIS BOOK

EMILY KILE
Burchfiel-Kile Enterprises
803 Dolly Parton Pkwy, Sevierville, TN

GORDON KLATT
Relay For Life
www.relayforlife.org/learn/dr-gordy-klatt

SOPHIA CONERLY
Relay For Life Of Sevier County
www.facebook.com/1relayforlifeofseviercounty

JORDAN PICKENS
ANN SUTTON BOWMAN
Captain Cancer Fighter
www.facebook.com/captaincancerfighter

DWINITA LOVEDAY
CATHY DOUGLAS
NOELLE AUSTIN
Tennessee State Bank
1375 Dolly Parton Parkway, Sevierville, TN

KELLY SNYDER
Preferred Pharmacy
1024 Middle Creek Rd #1, Sevierville, TN

MARC HIGHTOWER
Sky High Air Tours
134 Air Museum Way, Sevierville, TN

RANDY KING
www.mime4him.com/
www.facebook.com/mime4him

RON EMERY
Emery 5 & 10 General Store
131 The Island Drive, Pigeon Forge, TN

JONATHAN WRIGHT
Sign Master
110 Oak Cluster, Suite 1, Sevierville, TN

JENNIFER MacPHERSON-EVANS
CHRIS MacPHERSON
Sweet Fanny Adams Theater
www.sweetfannyadams.com

CASSIE JAMES-ARWOOD
CHRISTIN SMITH MATTHEWS
MACKIE JAMES
Shear Madness Beauty and Beyond
212 Collier Drive, Sevierville, TN

DR. TERRI DODGE
Principal at Sevierville Intermediate School
416 High Street, Sevierville, TN

ABOUT THE AUTHOR

Elyse Bruce does a lot of cool things. She's a musician, a composer, a singer-songwriter, a visual artist, an illustrator, a playwright, and an author as well as a mom.

She writes music, songs, short stories, novels and plays, when she isn't painting and photographing the neat things around her. She teaches songwriting and marketing classes at the college and university level, and leads workshops and seminars on a number of subjects.

Along with writing "The Missy Barrett Adventures" book series and "The Missy Barrett Conversations" book series, Elyse also writes the "Idiomation" book series and many other books.

She likes to create and promote new and exciting projects that engage, involve, and benefit as many people as possible. Just like Missy.

In her spare time, Elyse bakes chocolate chip cookies which she then generously shares with friends and family. Sometimes she even serves French Vanilla ice cream with chocolate sprinkles on top with those chocolate chip cookies!

OTHER MISSY BARRETT BOOKS

Missy Barrett Adventures
For Middle Grade Readers

Houston, We Have No Problems
Guess Where I Am, Mommy
The Secret Ingredient
Foiled Again
Free Range Hiking
Nailed It
Barnstormin'
The Living Statue

Missy Barrett Chapter Books
For All Ages

Roar Like A Lion
Fantastic Things
Pinwheels and Pearls

Missy Barrett Conversations
For All Ages

Barracudas and Impalas
Indians Live In Tipis

Missy Barrett Year In Review
For All Ages

The Year I Turned 8
The Year I Turned 9

Journals & Diaries
For All Ages

A Year Of Good Weeks

Novellas
For Tweens and Teens

Grand Theft: Cookie
featuring Missy Barrett

MISSY BARRETT ON SOCIAL MEDIA

Visit Missy Barrett's website at
www.missybarrett.com

Follow Missy Barrett's blog at
www.missybarrett.wordpress.com

Follow Missy Barrett on Facebook at
www.facebook.com/MissyBarrettFanPage

Follow Missy Barrett on Twitter at
www.twitter.com/glassonastick

Send Missy Barrett snail mail
at this address:

Missy Barrett
c/o Elyse Bruce
P.O. Box 6306
Sevierville, TN
37864